Acupressure Way of Health

acupressure way of health:
jin shin do

by iona teeguarden

japan publications, inc.

© 1978 in Japan by Iona Marsaa Teeguarden
Photographs by Ron Teeguarden and David Ford

Published by
JAPAN PUBLICATIONS, INC., Tokyo, Japan

Distributors:
United States: *Kodansha International/USA, Ltd., through Harper & Row, Publishers, Inc., 10 East 53rd Street, New York, New York 10022.* South America: *Harper & Row, Publishers, Inc., International Department.* Canada: *Fitzhenry & Whiteside Ltd., 150 Lesmill Road, Don Mills, Ontario M3B 2T6.* Mexico and Central America: *HARLA S. A. de C. V., Apartado 30–546, Mexico 4, D. F.* British Isles: *International Book Distributors Ltd., 66 Wood Lane End, Hemel Hempstead, Herts HPZ 4RG.* European Continent: *Boxerbooks, Inc., Limmatstrasse 111, 8031 Zurich.* Australia and New Zealand: *Book Wise (Australia) Pty. Ltd., 104–8 Sussex Street, Sydney 2000.* The Far East and Japan: *Japan Publications Trading Co., Ltd., 1–2–1, Sarugaku-cho, Chiyoda-ku, Tokyo 101.*

First edition: April 1978
Fifth printing: July 1982

ISBN 0–87040–421–0

Printed in U.S.A.

To New Age people everywhere;

To the Sages, past and present,
Who have pointed the Way to a New Age
Of compassion, love, and the joy of life;

And to my parents, who gave me
The gifts of life and love.

GRATITUDE

I would like to thank Michio Kushi and Herman Aihara, who introduced me to oriental health art philosophy; Jean-Claude Thomas Rholdes and Shui Wan Wu, who encouraged me in the study of acupuncture theory and philosophy; Mary Iino Burmeister, who introduced me to Jin Shin technique; Kok Yuen Leung, who has made much information on traditional theories and practices available to the West; Haruki Kato, who was a source of information as to Jiro Murai's spiritual and practical philosophies; Katsusuke Serizawa, M.D., who was a source of encouragement and inspiration; Sung Jin Park, who introduced me to basic Taoist yogic techniques; my clients and students, present and past, who have been my continuous inspiration; and Iajai, my Spirit Guide.

I would like to especially thank Ron Teeguarden, who has contributed many ideas and helped to give direction to the evolution of Jin Shin Do and to its growth in this country. Without his support in encouraging me to pursue acupressure seven years ago, in finding and introducing me to many great teachers and books, in helping me to communicate with Iajai in Japan, and throughout the growth of Jin Shin Do, this book would not have been possible.

PREFACE

The last century has seen Mankind riding an increasingly rapid spiral of activity. Productivity is the goal; constant animation the means. We modern, civilized human beings often find that we have forgotten how to relax our bodies and our minds. In an effort to shut out life's seemingly continuous roar of demands and dictates, pressures and problems, we have also shut out and lost touch with much of the beauty of our world.

The mental and physical tension resulting from this increasing cultural and personal hyper-activity have become almost inescapable. Simultaneously, we have to a large degree ignored the arts of physical culture, which would make us strong enough to deal with the pressures of a rather uptight world, and the arts of relaxation, or spiritual culture, which would make us calm and flexible enough. One task—or pleasure—of our age, then, is re-learning the ability to help ourselves and our friends, re-learning the simple skills of maintaining greater physical and emotional well-being.

A century ago, our ancestors were busy trying to import the material treasures of the Orient. Today, we find another kind of importing also going on—one anticipated by the most foresighted of our ancestors. This is the importation of oriental life-style treasures—methods used since ancient times to explore and develop our emotional, physical, and spiritual beings. These methods can help provide a necessary balance to our recently acquired sedentary life-styles and intellectual emphases. They also include amazing techniques for helping us release tension and deal with pressure or frustration, worry or depression.

Surprisingly, our needs today are not so different from those of the ancient oriental civilizations. We read in the *Nei Ching,* or *Yellow Emperor's Classic of Internal Medicine*, written around the fourth century B. C.:

"In former times man lived among birds, beasts, and reptiles; he worked, moved, and stirred in order to avoid and to escape the cold and darkness, and he sought a dwelling into which he could flee from the heat. Within him there were no family ties which bound him with love; on the outside there were no officials who could guide out and correct his physical appearance. Into this tranquil and peaceful era evil influences could not penetrate deeply . . .

"But the present world is a different one. Grief, calamity, and evil cause inner bitterness, while the body receives wounds from the outside; moreover there is neglect against the laws of the four seasons, there is disobedience and rebellion, and there are those who violate the customs of what is proper during the cold of Winter and the heat of Summer. Reprimands are in vain. Evil influences strike from early morning until late at night; they injure the five viscera, the bones and marrow within the body, and externally they injure the mind and reduce its intelligence, and they also injure the muscles and the flesh...”[1]

Therefore, in ancient Japan, China, and Korea, many health arts were developed in order to balance the body and mind. These included exercise patterns, meditation techniques, martial arts, and acupressure (finger pressure) methods. All are based on the same fundamental philosophy and are designed to strengthen and energize the body and mind. All are treasures, which now we in the West can also use to achieve happier and healthier states of being.

Acupuncture, or needle insertion, was traditionally one of the methods used by oriental therapists and doctors. Acupressure, while it has been and is now being used by therapists and doctors, primarily was a folk art belonging to the common people. Acupuncture is about 5000 years old, with written records of its practice dating from the fifth century B. C. Yet acupressure is even more ancient, for it is from the simple finger-pressure techniques that acupuncture was evolved.

The continued use and development of acupressure by laymen has been encouraged by both ancient and modern oriental doctors, who place great emphasis on preventative medicine and on practical methods of maintaining well-being. The *Nei Ching* records that “the sages did not treat those who were already ill; they instructed those who were not yet ill. They did not want to rule those who were already rebellious; they guided those who were not yet rebellious. To administer medicines to diseases which have already developed and to suppress revolts which have already developed is comparable to the behavior of persons who begin to dig a well after they become thirsty, and of those who begin to cast weapons after they have already engaged in battle. Would these actions not be too late?”[2] Perhaps our answer might be, “Not always.” Perhaps we are not always omniscient and omnipotent enough to never develop dis-ease and never need medical help. But even if we begin in small ways to develop and maintain well-being, we are at least starting to dig the well, beginning to quell the revolt. ‘A thousand miles’ journey begins from the spot under one’s feet.”[3]

Acupuncture requires a long-term dedication and a great deal of study before its practice, because it involves the insertion of needles into the human body. Acupressure was traditionally regarded as a very helpful requisite for the training acupuncturist, because it develops a feeling for locating pressure points and enables the immediate practical use of both basic and advanced theory and philosophy. Acupressure was itself one of the traditional trades: it was also used to some degree by most of the

---

[1]*Nei Ching*, from section 13.
[2]*Ibid.*, from section 2.
[3]*Tao Teh Ching*, from Chapter LXIII.

common people, because it is relatively easy to learn and completely safe
to practice.

The particular acupressure technique used in Jin Shin Do derives partially from an art called "Jin Shin Jitsu." Based on traditional Japanese
acupressure methods, as well as meditation techniques, Jin Shin Jitsu was
developed by Jiro Murai in Japan during the thirties through early sixties
of this century. Jin Shin Do acupressure stays close to traditional theories
and techniques, while directing its practices towards the needs of our culture and age. Its acupressure patterns are derived from acupuncture theory
and from the practices of many generous acupuncture masters, as well as
from research on and study of Jin Shin Do and other acupressure methods
here and in Japan. In order to work on the whole person as effectively as
possible, Jin Shin Do practitioners also use basic Taoist yogic techniques
(breathing, meditation, and exercise methods) and traditional dietary principles.

Jin Shin Do can be practiced on several different levels. It emphasizes
developing and maintaining well-being, rather than concentrating on a
symptomatic approach. It aims at a deep release and rejuvenation, through
which the higher, or psychic, centers can be opened. Jin Shin Do may be
studied as a way of understanding basic oriental philosophy and of
increasing our own boby-mind awareness. It may also be studied as a way
of helping one's family and friends, or even as a part-time or full-time
profession after sufficient study and practice.[1]

In this book, I have tried to present traditional oriental philosophy and
health practices in a way which might be readily accessible to this age. I
hope that it may serve as an introduction to the veritable treasure-house
that is the ancient oriental Way, and help many people to incorporate these
magical and powerful oriental health arts into their own life-styles.

Sometimes these teachings, or parts of them, have been kept secret, either
for fear of spreading them to persons who would mis-use them, or else in
order to maintain a profession (such as that of acupuncturist) for one's
sons and one's son's sons. We must always be very grateful to those oriental teachers and masters who, seeing the great needs of this materialistic age,
have chosen to give freely of their knowledge and wisdom.

The Yellow Emperor said, "When the spiritual powers are passed on
and transmitted they can no longer turn back; and when they turn

[1] As finger pressure, Jin Shin Do acupressure falls into the western category of massage.
It is not a medical practice, and should not be interpreted as such, though it can certain-
ly serve as a helpful adjunct to medical or psychological therapy. Because Jin Shin Do
acupressure is like western massage only in that it uses the human touch to work on the
(usually clothed) body, the words "treatment" and "treater" are generally used rather
than the words "massage" and "masseur" or "masseuse." The words "treatment" and
"treater" (or, alternately, "practitioner") are not meant to in any way convey or carry
any medical meaning or interpretation. Jin Shin Do is, quite simply, a helping art, and
Jin Shin Do-ists are but helpers.

back they cannot be transmitted, and then their moving powers are lost to the universe. In order to fulfill destiny man should go beyond that which is near at hand and consider it as trifling. One should make public upon tablets of jade that which was hidden and concealed in treasuries and storehouses, to study it from early dawn until night, and thus make known the precious mechanism of the universe."[1]

Iona Marsaa Teeguarden

Tokyo, Los Angeles, and North Dakota
July 1976–August 1977

---

[1] *Nei Ching,* from section 19.

CONTENTS

1. THE CHAPTER OF CONCEPTION

One simple way in which we should be able to help ourselves and our friends and family is through the power of the human touch. We are all born with this power, with the ability to help release tension and re-vitalize the body energy through touch. In spite of years of chaotic life-styles induced by the pressures of modern times, this magical power is never completely atrophied; neither is our need for touch ever eliminated.

In ancient times, almost everyone in the Orient knew how to use some form of acupressure to help their family and friends through the power of touch. Acupressure—literally "finger pressure"—is very simple to learn and practice. Use of this and related oriental health arts can help us recover the ability to help ourselves to happier, healthier, and freer lives.

Although everyone has this amazing power of the touch, its release needs a catalyst. The most powerful one is love or compassion. That is why Jin Shin Do, which revolves around a traditional Japanese acupressure art, literally means "The Way of the Compassionate Spirit." Compassion is the key to helping others and to helping ourselves.

Through the power of the touch in Jin Shin Do acupressure, we can experience a new and wonderful state of energic balance —a balance which pervades the whole of our physical, emotional, mental, and spiritual states of being.[1] By giving and receiving acupressure treatments, we also become increasingly aware of our own conditions and of our body's vital energies. We begin to notice that certain environments and situations initiate or increase our feeling of tension and imbalance, while other environments and situations induce feelings of happiness and well-being. Through this increased awareness of our own internal body-mind unity, and of the unity between the individual and the environment, we can learn to maintain the balanced state that we experience through the acupressure treatment.

What is health? What is dis-ease? The traditional oriental definition of health is not merely the absence of dis-ease, but beyond that a state of balance and a feeling of well-being. "When the forces of the body work in mutual harmony there will be life (or vitality); when they associate with each other but do not blend illness will result."[2] Behind all traditional oriental therapeutic practices and health arts is the principle that health is balance and dis-ease a lack of balance of the vital energy.

---

[1]Because the art of acupressure is relatively new to this country, its English vocabulary is still in the formative stage: Meridian, for example, is the accepted term to denote the flow lines, even though this meaning does not appear in most dictionaries. There is no word, however, that denotes that aspect of our being which is comprised of the vital life energy of the ki. Rather than continue to use "energy" and "energetic" as poor substitutes, I suggest that we coin the term "energic" to use as an adjective meaning "of or relating to the energy aspect of being," just as nineteenth century physicists introduced the term "etheric" to mean "of or pertaining to ether." Thus we would speak of energic balance, in the same way that we speak of emotional, mental or spiritual states.

[2]Nei Ching, from section 20.

14

This vital energy, the "Ki," is similar to but more subtle than electromagnetic energy. We receive this energy in several ways. There is pre-natal ki—that which we receive from our father and mother before birth, and also post-natal ki—that which we receive mainly through our food and breath after we are born. Running through the body in orderly pathways called "meridians" and "channels," this ki nourishes and defends the body. It is the most primal energy of the body, sustaining and coordinating all its activities.

Remaining centered, maintaining a state of balance, is difficult under the pressures of modern civilization. So many social and material forces constantly influence us, confusing and complicating almost every aspect of our lives. Today more than ever, we need to recover and use the simple wisdom of the ancients.

What is Jin Shin Do?

Designed to replenish and harmonize the vital energy of the body and to balance and strengthen the body and the spirit, Jin Shin Do is a correlation of ancient oriental health arts.[1] It is a healthway which revolves around an amazing acupressure technique, and also includes other traditional oriental life arts such as breathing and meditation methods, physical exercise systems, and traditional dietary principles. Important as these are, individually and as a whole, the most important aspect of Jin Shin Do is a basic understanding without which any technique is an empty husk. The understanding of basic oriental philosophy cannot be separated from the study of practical techniques for, in its origin and development, any oriental health art is firmly rooted in this basic philosophy or view of life.

The name "Jin Shin Do" describes some of the most fundamental principles of oriental philosophy as related to the health arts. Its

characters are:

仁　　　神　　　道
Jin　　　Shin　　　Do
(Compassion) (Spirit) (Tao, Way)

Jin—Compassion

The first character, Jin (or Jen—Chinese), is the only prerequisite for the study of Jin Shin Do. Jin means compassion or benevolence— the magic key that unlocks the true power of our inner spirit. Without compassion for ourselves, the spiral of personal development is constantly impeded by hypercriticism and its children—doubt, insecurity, and negativism. Without compassion for others, any body-mind work done to help them is but mechanics—a set of technical adjustments having only superficial effect and powerless to reach the spiritual core of the other's being. Compassion is the arrow sent from our spiritual center, carrying not only our own spirit but also the spirit of the other into the high and clear realms of freedom and joy.

What creates compassion? On the one hand, reflection on our own frailties and difficulties; experience of the passions—joy and sorrow, fear and anger, love and grief; and thus awareness of the human condition. On the other hand, seeing that "those who are at the point of an abyss feel as though their hands were in the grip of a tiger; at that time their energy and care are not devoted to the care of all creation."[2] When dis-ease grips us, our energy is directed internally towards the care of ourselves; we are usually not able to direct our energy externally to really care for our family, our friends, and all creation.

[1]Pronounced Jin (as in "trip"), Shin (as in "trip"), Do (as in "flow").
[2]*Nei Ching*, from section 25.

Shin—Spirit

The second character, Shin (or Shen—Chinese), means Spirit. It also carries the meaning of "extending" or "creating." Shin dwells in the human heart and is the master or creator of the physical and emotional natures, ruling all the activities of ki in both body and mind. Shin is in fact Tao within us, or God within us. It is the divinely-inspired part of man. From a balanced Shin come the emotions of joy and love, expressed in free laughter and warm smiles.

Like a glass, Shin can be clear and sparkling, or foggy and clouded. When it is clouded, our perception is distorted. We perceive Spirit as being "ours"—belonging to ourselves and separate from the rest of creation. Because we lose touch with the Tao, we try to possess Spirit, to brand it with our personal trademark. We may accept the necessity of flowing with the constant changes of our world—but we insist on a boat painted our favorite color, our name emblazoned on its side. Thus we confuse Spirit with ego, turning our natural drive to self-growth into excessive self-preoccupation. We take ourselves too seriously. This ordinary consciousness is the cloud distorting our perception, alienating us from Nature or Tao. At birth or in the course of life, this clouded perception overwhelms our original Spirit—our primal or spiritual consciousness.

When we take the cloths of self-awareness —reflection, release, and meditation—to clean and polish the glass, we find that ordinary consciousness has vanished. Just as in looking through a dirty or foggy glass we may "see" something that is not really there, so in looking through a cloudy Shin we may perceive an ego-centered "reality" that is not real at all, or is but part of the real.

What do we see instead? What is the clear Shin? The unfoggy Shin, or Shen, is our Spirit in tune with nature, seeing the oneness

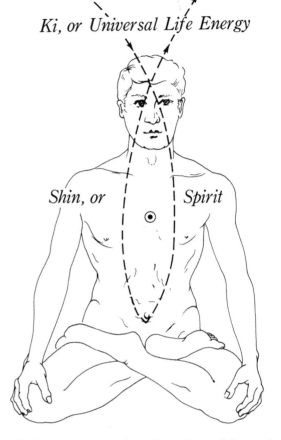

Ki, or Universal Life Energy

Shin, or　　　*Spirit*

of all things, accepting the universal flow of change and reveling in the cosmic play. "Let me discuss Shen, the spirit," says Ch'i Po to the Yellow Emperor. "What is the spirit? The spirit cannot be heard with the ear. The eye must be brilliant of perception and the heart must be open and attentive, and then the spirit is suddenly revealed through one's own consciousness. It cannot be expressed through the mouth; only the heart can express all that can be looked upon. If one pays close attention, one may suddenly know it, but one can just as suddenly lose this knowledge. But Shen, the spirit, becomes clear to man as though the wind has blown away the cloud. Therefore one speaks of it as the spirit."[1]

---

[1] *Nei Ching*, from section 26.

Shin (or Shen) resides in the heart and is associated with the upper chest center (the heart, chakra). It rules the physical energies, harmonizes the emotions, and guides all the workings of the intellect and the will.

Jin Shin Do is the way of the compassionate spirit; it is also one way to the compassionate spirit. As we manifest compassion, such as through the touch in Jin Shin Do acupressure, our spirits become progressively clearer. The ability to absorb and use the universal energy, or ki, increases. Shin is strengthened so that its true desires—the dictates of our inner hearts—are revealed to us. When we experience freedom of the spirit, when the spiritual consciousness rules, even briefly, the spiritual attitude begins to be transmuted. The emotions become more balanced, the physical energies are strengthened, and there is harmony between the body and mind.

Do—Tao or Way

The third character, Do or Tao (Chinese), literally means Way—the Way followed by all the Universe including Man. The word "Tao" is used in as many different ways as the word "God," but is not quite the same as what we usually mean by God.[1] The most fundamental principle of all oriental philosophy, Tao is ultimate reality, the way in which Nature works. Lao Tzu, in the ancient classic of oriental philosophy called the "Tao Teh Ching," says Tao is the "origin of heaven and earth," the "Door of all essence."

Lao Tzu's first words about the Tao, the opening words of the Tao Teh Ching, are "The Tao that can be expressed is not the eternal Tao . . . " The Tao is absolute and unlimited, whereas words are relative and limited. Words are boxes which cannot contain entire visions of the Tao, but only parts of that vision. Words also involve at least two different sets of connotations and

associations—those of the author or speaker and those of the reader or listener. Thus, especially when talking of the Tao, we must attempt to feel the spirit of the words, using words as brush strokes with which we try to paint, as clearly as possible, a picture of the whole thinking-feeling-being context of the thing or thought at hand.

Here is Lao Tzu's word-picture of the Tao:

> *"There is a thing inherent and natural,*
> *Which existed before heaven and earth.*
> *Motionless and fathomless,*
> *It stands alone and never changes;*
> *It pervades everywhere and never becomes exhausted.*
> *It may be regarded as the Mother of the Universe.*
> *I do not know its name.*
> *If I am forced to give it a name,*
> *I call it Tao, and I name it as supreme (far-reaching).*
> *Supreme means going on;*
> *Going on means going far;*
> *Going far means returning.*
> *Therefore Tao is supreme; heaven is supreme; earth is supreme; and man is also supreme. There are in the universe four things supreme, and man is one of them.*
> *Man follows the laws of earth;*
> *Earth follows the laws of heaven;*
> *Heaven follows the laws of Tao;*
> *Tao follows the laws of its intrinsic nature."*[2]

This means that Tao includes everything that is—and everything that is not, too. Both heaven and earth, day and night, light and dark, spirit and body—all participate in, or

[1]Throughout the text it is the Japanese term that is generally used, and the Chinese that is indicated. I have chosen to use the Chinese Tao, however, since it is used almost universally. (Tao is pronounced dow, and rhymes with "how.")
[2]*Tao Teh Ching*, Chapter XXV.

are, the Tao. The movement of the Tao is continuous "going far" and "returning"—continuous cyclic change. This is the order of the macrocosm (the universe) and of the microcosm (man). The vision of the Tao impels man to begin to harmonize his life with the music of the spheres, to be aware of and flow with the changes that compose the journey of life. "Those who are in harmony are like an echo . . . they follow (their way) Tao, and need neither demons nor gods, for they are free and independent."[1]

Thus Tao also has a more personal meaning of the way or path to clearer realization of our Tao-ness. Just as the way to an earthly place may be found along many different paths, all leading there, so the Tao includes many different individual ways—as many ways as there are people on the planet. Once we have found our own individual way, the path of our true spirit, we must be grateful and maintain this way as long as it has soul for us. But many times we find one way, put a box around it, and then think it is The Only Way for ourselves and for everyone. The Tao Way is not exclusive. It sees behind form and language to the necessary unity of all truth. The Tao Way is tolerant of and encourages any path that reveals to anyone his essential Tao-ness.

AN OLD STORY

A man was journeying up a mountain.
He looked around and saw others going
A different way, even
A different direction.

"Fools!" he thought, "They are going the
Wrong way."

The man kept journeying until,
Years later, he reached the top—
It was a very high mountain.
And then, he saw
Those other Fools.
They were on top of the mountain too.

How Does Jin Shin Do Work?

The various Jin Shin Do techniques are ways of becoming still enough to really be aware, to really see and hear our world. They are ways of becoming balanced and centered—through acupressure release, meditation, breathing techniques, movement, and diet—so that we can experience the joy of internal and external unity.

So much of the time we spend our lives just looking at and listening to our world, allowing our particular mental and emotional sets to filter our perception of the world so that we do not really see and hear. In effect, by our own thought and feeling habit patterns we censor ourselves, allowing ourselves to absorb some things but not others. The more rigid our patterns become, the more spontaneity we lose. We habitually react, rather than spontaneously act. We are missing something. We are missing some pieces of the puzzle, because we are filtering them out. We are allowing the filters of our perceptions, feelings, and thoughts—our ordinary consciousness—to cover our original, spiritual consciousness. Because of these filters, these addictions of Shin or Spirit, we are missing the joyous awareness of the free Spirit. We all, at some point, choose to filter or not to filter. But we are all inherently free.

We have a wide choice of filters: worry, greed, fear, anger, and sorrow, to name a few. All of these emotional imbalances reflect or are reflected in mental patterns, and also in physical patterns. Just as imbalanced posture and movement habits will affect specific areas and be affected by specific areas of the body, so too the various emotional imbalances are each reflected in muscular tension and armoring at certain body areas. This armoring tends

---

[2]*Nei Ching*, from section 25.

to continue and re-create the specific emotional imbalances, obstructing our clear vision of Tao by filtering out parts of the here-and-now.

We can begin the process of shedding self-destructive filters by working at either end of the body-mind spectrum. We can begin with body-work, releasing physical armoring and re-balancing ourselves structurally and energically. Or we can begin with mind-work, with mental, emotional, and spiritual release and re-balancing. According to traditional oriental philosophy, there is really no separation between the body and mind; they are completely inter-related. By working on one aspect of our being, the other is necessarily affected. But in most effectively working on either aspect, the other must be considered. The combination of acupressure with other traditional health practices, as in Jin Shin Do, was thus a traditional method of facilitating the release of old self-destructive patterns and aiding the establishment of new balance in both the body and the mind.

A wholistic way, Jin Shin Do can include:

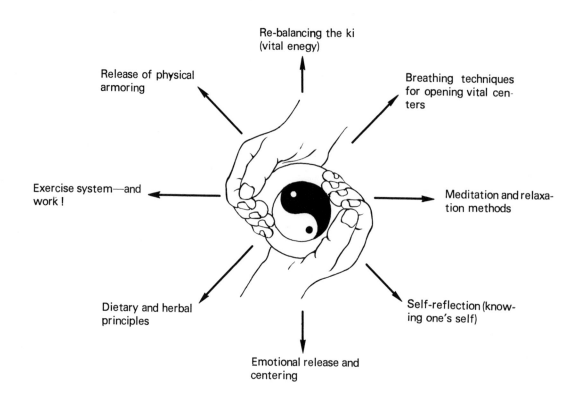

Re-balancing the ki
(vital enegy)

Release of physical
armoring

Breathing techniques
for opening vital cen-
ters

Exercise system—and
work !

Meditation and relaxa-
tion methods

Dietary and herbal
principles

Self-reflection (know-
ing one's self)

Emotional release and
centering

Jin Shin Do acupressure and other techniques are based on traditional oriental philosophy, theory, and practice. These arts have been used and developed for centuries, so in a sense they are very sophisticated and highly-evolved. But they are also, at their base, very simple and easy to learn. Each age, and each person, must absorb this traditional wisdom and then use and develop it according to present needs and conditions. That is to say, each must follow his or her own way.

Each person can find in the traditional health arts of Jin Shin Do at least an enhancement of his or her own way, and an opening to other ways. Many who study these arts may find even more than this—a Way which will open their paths in life and through which they can continuously develop. This is possible only through absorbing these ancient wisdoms and then making them one's own, bringing these ancient principles and techniques to life, or re-creating them, through reflection and use. Such creativity proceeds from the Shin, or Spirit. In its spontaneity it reflects the Tao.

At this time, when Mankind stands tottering at the change of the ages, with many wondering if in fact the New Age of Man and its unviolent heralding are even possible, the planet has great need for compassionate men and compassionate women and their Ways. We must awaken to our essential oneness, to the oneness of the people with the planet, and to the need to join together in evolving the condition of both. There is much to be done on the external or ecological scale, and much also on the internal or personal. By releasing ourselves from rigidities and blocks, by becoming centered in our Spirits and balanced in our energy flows, and by helping others to become more released and balanced, we can help our planet as well. If we can realize (literally, make real) the principle that health and happiness mean harmony with Nature, and with our Inner Natures, then planetary and personal conditions will necessarily improve.

There is no separation between macrocosm and microcosm; neither is there any separation within the microcosm. This unity of all things—of universe and man, and of man's body and mind—is the most basic premise of all oriental philosophy. It underlies the conception of all traditional techniques for evolving the body-mind condition. The planet is one with its people, and the people's actions are harmonious or not, according to their internal states of being. There are no panaceas, no universal rules for harmonizing the body and mind. But there are techniques we can learn to assist us in tuning in to our inner Spirits and learning to balance our internal states of being.

The Spiral of Time Change

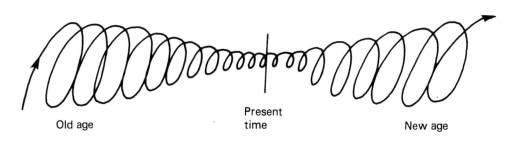

Old age   Present time   New age

The points of change between the ages are the times of greatest intensity. The present is such a time. The spiral of change is revolving very quickly; things are changing rapidly in almost every aspect of life. To see change going on at this time is fairy easy. To flow with the constant changes is more difficult—and more necessary, if we are not to be overwhelmed by their rapidity.

2. THE GOVERNING CHAPTER

Two fundamental principles are the basis of all oriental therapeutic and health art philosophy. If we become aware of, understand, and use just these two principles, then all the theories behind oriental health arts—no matter how vague or complex they may seem at first sight—can be readily learned and competently used. In fact, all other principles, though fascinating and important, are only correlates of these two.

The two governing principles are: 1) the dynamic yin-yang principle, and 2) the principle of ki, or vital energy. These ancient oriental principles were expressed in writing as early as the first half of the first millennium B.C.—almost three thousand years ago—in the *I Ching*, or Book of Changes. They were discussed in the ancient classic of oriental philosophy, the *Tao Teh Ching*, written around the fourth century B.C., and their therapeutic implications were expressed in detail in the monumental *Nei Ching*, or *Yellow Emperor's Classic of Internal Medicine*, written around the same period. This classic is still a fundamental textbook for the modern acupuncturist or acupressurist, and these two principles are still the basic premise of all oriental health arts.

The Tao of Bodywork

The great Taoist sage Lao Tzu describes the existence and nature of these two fundamental principles very simply:

> "*The Tao begets the One,*
> *The One begets the two,*
> *The two beget the three, and*

> *The three beget the ten thousand things.*
> *All things are backed by the Shade (yin)*
> *And faced by the Light (yang),*
> *And harmonized by the immaterial Breath (ch'i).*"[1]

What does this mean? The Tao is the primordial, ultimate, and infinite Source. It becomes the One, a unity of forces, in order to manifest itself. "All things by Unity have come into existence."[2] The Tao remains the One, united, even as, like the lowly amoeba, it draws apart into its front and back. Making itself into cosmic playmates, the One thus separates into two forces: the yin and the yang.

What are these primal "two"? What are yin and yang? They are simply words used to describe the two faces of Unity, the opposite but complementary forces that we find in every being and in every process. The most primal manifestations of yin and yang are heaven or space (yang) and earth or form (yin), also day or light (yang) and night or darkness (yin). "In the beginning God created the heavens and the earth . . . and God separated the light from the darkness."[3]

Yin and yang do not exist independently of each other, either in our universe or in our minds. It is impossible to conceive of an earth not surrounded and supported by the heavens; on the other hand, even in outer space matter exists, though its distribution is

---

[1] *Tao Teh Ching*, from Chapter XLII.
[2] *Ibid.*, from Chapter XXXIX.
[3] *The Bible* (Oxford edition), Genesis I, 1 and 4.

rather less dense than within a planet or earth. If there were no darkness, we would not have the concept of light, for there would be nothing to compare it with. Yin and yang exist relative to each other.

Basically, yin is the passive force; yang is active. Yin is receptive; yang is assertive. All things contain both yin and yang, though one force may dominate the other. "All things are backed by the yin, and faced by the yang." When our life-styles are full of activity and busy-ness, the yang force is dominant. When our lives are quieter, with more time for relaxation, the yin force is dominant in our life-styles. The point of yin-yang philosophy is that both forces are essential in our universe and in our personal lives.

What we need to learn is the art of attaining and maintaining a balance between the two. For example, when the yang force dominates our life-styles to an extreme, we may experience tension; when the yin force is too dominant, we may experience lethargy and weakness. The ideal is to be yang and yin, active and passive, according to circumstances: to be able to tense our muscles or activate our minds, and then to also relax our muscles and quiet our minds when the need for activity has passed.

We have seen the Tao making the One, and the One making the two. So the etheric curtain opens and the cosmic play begins. The two—yin and yang—interact like protagonists on an earthly stage, or like friends communicating with each other. Between them a vibration is created. It is a very subtle, etheric, high vibration—the basic energy of the universe, the vital life force. Similar to but subtler than electro-magnetic energy, it is called ki in Japan, chi (or ch'i) in China, qi in Korea, prana in India, rlun in Tibet, orgone energy in the works of Wilhelm Reich, and bioplasma or vital energy in the terms of modern western scientists.

Ki is all around us and within us, always changing, following the natural laws of yin and yang. We are like fish living in an ocean of ki. We are supported and nourished by this vital life energy, yet we are usually not aware of its existence and importance.

Western scientists analyze the material world, dividing it into finer and finer, smaller and smaller particles, only to discover, in the ultimate insights of the most advanced research, that way down deep inside the tunnel, at the very core of what is, we find energy. This is the ultimate simplicity, and it was the starting point of all oriental therapies and health arts.

Energy preceds matter, just as thought or feeling preceds action. Ki is the basic life energy, and ki is governed in its manifestations by the workings of the dynamic yin-yang principle. Therefore, as Lao Tzu said, the three—the yin force, the yang force, and ki—create the ten thousand things.

According to oriental philosophy, all living things contain ki. The harmony of the ki—its yin-yang balance—is necessary for the well-functioning of any living thing. Therefore, all the ten thousand things are "harmonized by the immaterial breath (ch'i)." It is through control of the ch'i or ki that harmony or balance between the yin and the yang can most easily be developed. This is a process of centering, of finding the "Great Ridge-Pole" (Tai Ch'i) around which the polar opposites revolve harmoniously.

Yin and Yang, a Spiral of Change

We can use the yin-yang principle as just a new and different analytical tool, categorizing all things according to yin and yang[1]. Though such descriptions can help to expand our

---

[1]During different times and in different areas of the Orient, yin and yang have had different pronuncia-

awareness of our world, they are but static intellectual concepts unless we add understanding of the dynamic nature of yin and yang. Yin and yang are, most importantly, a way of describing change, a way of seeing and feeling the rhythms of life.

Though the art or science of yin-yang was most highly developed in the ancient Orient, yin-yang thinking is basic to many traditional cultures, for change—the existence and interaction of polarities—is basic to life. Today, the ancient yin-yang philosophy which was so fundamental to traditional oriental philosophers and therapists is echoed in the modern science of biological rhythms. "Invisible rhythms underlie most of what we assume to be constant in ourselves and the world around us," begins a report on biological rhythms by the National Institute of Mental Health. "Life is in constant flux, but the change is not chaotic. The rhythmic nature of earth life is, perhaps, its most usual yet overlooked property . . . Night follows day. Seasons change. The tides ebb and flow. These various rhythms are also seen in animals and man. We, too, change, growing sleepy at night and restlessly active by day. We, too, exhibit the rhythmic undulations of our planet."[1]

If we look at the yin-yang symbol itself, we see that it is not a static symbol at all but rather a flowing and vital one, illustrating continual rhythmic change. Yin is symbolized by the black (or sometimes green) portion, representing that which is passive, receptive, yielding, dark, cold. Yang is symbolized by the white (or sometimes red) portion, representing that which is active, assertive, firm,

bright, warm. These are the two vital forces of life, the two basic tendencies of all creation. They are like the warp and woof threads of life, together weaving the fabric of existence with all of its varied and interesting patterns and hues.

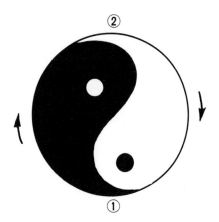

Starting at ① on the above yin-yang symbol, we see that here the dark, or yin, portion of the circle is at its smallest. As we follow the circle around in a clockwise direction, yin is gradually becoming bigger until it is the largest at ②. At that point, it begins to change into yang, which here is at its smallest. Continuing to follow the circle around in the clockwise direction, we see the white, or yang, portion now gradually becoming larger until back at ① it is at its largest and changes back into yin.

If we continue to follow the circle round and round, we see that the process of change described by the yin-yang symbol is not just a circle, but a cycle of constant change from yin to yang to yin to yang. But this does not mean that existence is a futile round of

tions. "Yin" and "Yang" are the words most commonly used in the West; therefore we retain these although "yin" (pronounced "een") and "yo-o" (pronounced as in yoga) are presently used in Japan. The most usual pronunciation of yin and yang is the Chinese pronunciation, in which the "y" is enunciated in "yin." Yin is thus pronounced "yēn."

"Yang" is pronounced with the soft vowel sound of "yawn" and not the more nasal sound of "bang."

[1]*Biological Rhythms in human and Animal Physiology*, by Gay Luce, Dover Publications, Inc., New York, 1971. First published as Public Health Service Publication.

24

meaningless change in which we are trapped. Basic to all oriental philosophy is an accepting or appreciative faith in the order of the universe, including both nature and human nature. "The great virtue as manifested is but following Tao," says Lao Tzu. ". . . This essence (Tao) being invariably true, there is faith in it."[1] Such faith brings peace and tranquility, for "where Tao is, equilibrium is."[2] Faith in the Tao results naturally from seeing the Tao; it is not an artificial, forced belief. "The honouring of Tao and the esteem of (the great) virtue are done, not by command, but always of their own accord."[3]

Tao is the "great virtue;" its Way is inherently "virtuous" in the sense of a direction towards the Greatest Good. How does the Tao act? How does it manifest the greatest virtue? "The Tao of heaven is to lessen the redundant and fill up the insufficient."[4]

What is not needed is taken away; what is needful comes. There is no concept here of a battle between the forces of righteousness and the forces of evil. "The Tao of heaven does not contend; yet it surely wins the victory."[5]

Faith in the Tao is faith not just in cycles but in a spiral of change, for a spiral is a cycle with direction. The Tao pervades all things and gives being to all things. Because of their essential Tao-ness, there is a direction to the continuous change of all things. This direction is not exactly a divine purpose, but rather a constant drawing closer to the Tao, the Source, like a child to its mother. This is true both of nature and of human nature, for both are manifestations of the Tao. "The Tao is ever inactive, and yet there is nothing it does not do. If princes and kings could keep to it, all things would themselves become developed."[6]

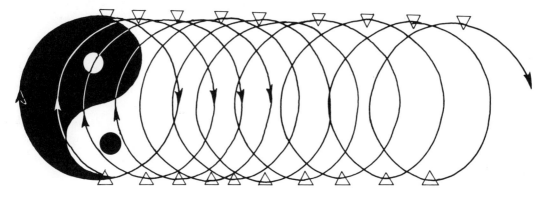

Yin and Yang: A Spiral of Change

The Taoist, the person who follows the Tao Way, does not try to force a "good" direction onto the development of things. Rather, he is concerned with developing himself, uncovering his original spirit, his Tao nature. Lao Tzu says, "I alone am different from others. But I value seeking sustenance from the Mother."[7]

This is the highest development of selfishness—valuing the search for internal clarity and nourishment. We are all inherently self-

ish, for we all share a common desire for the greatest happiness. Even while we are helping others, we act in ways which we hope or know will directly or indirectly make us

[1] *Tao Teh Ching*, from Chapter XXI.
[2] *Ibid.*, from Chapter XVIII.
[3] *Ibid.*, from Chapter LI.
[4] *Ibid.*, from Chapter LXXVII.
[5] *Ibid.*, from Chapter LXXIII.
[6] *Ibid.*, from Chapter XXXVII.
[7] *Ibid.*, from Chapter XX.

happier. The happiness we seek cannot be attained only by tuning in to our inner Natures, but neither can it be attained only by tuning in to other human natures. We must be free to do both—to be both passive and active.

Without being directed towards our own growth, we can hardly facilitate that of others. Yet we are all somewhat ashamed of selfishness. It is important to realize that to be always unselfish and never selfish is an impossible and unnecessary burden. As we see and validate our own inner desires, we begin to feel the forces that all people share. True compassion and love for others is born, and we begin to respond more spontaneously and directly to others.

Why are we afraid of selfishness? Why do we fear just doing what we really want to do, or letting others do what they really want to do? Because we do not truly have faith in Nature, or in human nature. We fear the inherent nature of the world and of mankind.

When there is faith in the Tao, and when man patterns his life on its Way, the Tao naturally works through man. When we forget the Tao within us, we must rely solely on our own individual powers, for we have cut ourselves off from "The Force," or the Universal Way. This is a great pressure to put on one's self! We would be very resentful if someone else put such a large pressure on us, forced us to assume such a great burden. And in fact we are inwardly resentful of this pressure. We are inwardly frustrated, worried, and anxious as much from our own assumption of this immense personal responsibility as from anything which others have done to us.

When we relax our self-seriousness and accept the universal flow of things, that flow begins to work through us. By accepting Tao within us, we allow Tao to work through us. And very interesting things begin to happen. This is an amazingly freeing philosophy,

for it removes the intense pressure of trying to ourselves establish the virtuous Way. It says that Way, that ultimate virtue, already exists: we have only to accept our participation in it. Yet this is freedom within the Tao, not freedom from the Tao. "What is against Tao will soon come to an end."

The spontaneous response to freedom of the Spirit is laughter. Laughter is the expression of organic relief as the tension of extreme self-pressure slips away. Laughter or warm smiles are the physical manifestation of the individual's joy at merging with his Source, like the laughter of a child running to his mother. Thus, as Michio Kushi, a leading oriental philosopher and teacher, says: "The difference between the Free Man and the Saint is that the free man is more humorous!"

Examples of Yin-Yang Change

All art, all work, all of life manifests the cycle of change described by the yin-yang symbol. This symbol basically illustrates the cycle of change between the yang and the yin—activity and passivity. It also shows us that this change is a gradual one, from little yang to big yang to little yin to big yin back to little yang etc.

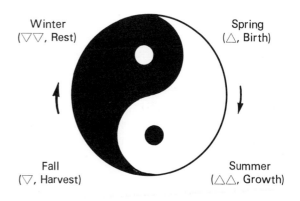

One of the most primary examples of yin-yang change is that of the seasons. Summer, the hottest season and the time of growth in Nature, is the most yang season. Winter, the coldest season and the time of rest or hibernation in Nature, is the most yin season. Spring, usually a warm season and also the time of birth and regeneration, is yang; fall, usually a cooler season and the time of harvest, is yin. Summer changes into fall, fall into winter, winter into spring, and spring into summer, continuously.

In our activities, we tend to reflect the cyclic changes of the seasons. We, too, feel a sense of regeneration during the spring, when all of nature is giving birth. During the summer, as the plants and crops and young animals are growing, we too feel like being active physically. During the fall, as the crops are maturing and being harvested, the leaves turning color and dropping from the trees, we begin to turn to quieter pursuits. And in the winter, we spend more time indoors, relaxing, or talking, or thinking.

In order to maintain a balance with the environment, our bodies respond to this cycle of nature by becoming more yin during extremes of yang (heat) and more yang during extremes of yin (cold). On hot days, the pores of our skin open so that the body perspires and is cooled. On cold days, the pores close and the blood vessels contract, conserving the body heat. This and other types of body adaptability can be encouraged by our lifestyle, which should be in tune with the changes of our environment.

The Yellow Emperor said, "Covered by Heaven and supported by Earth, all creation together in its most complete perfection is planned for the greatest achievement: Man. Man lives on the breath of Heaven and Earth, and he achieves perfection through the laws of the four seasons. The ruler as well as the masses share their utmost desire: the wish for a perfect body."[1]

How do we follow the laws of the four seasons? During the summer, we intuitively assist the cooling of our bodies by eating a more yin diet—more fruits and vegetables, less salt and more liquids. We wear lighter clothing and seek cooler, more yin environments after being out in the sun. During the winter, we are instead attracted to more yang foods—more cooked foods, more grains, perhaps animal food, and less liquids—to help warm our bodies. We wear warmer clothing and seek warmer environments—the proverbial fire in the hearth—after braving the cold.

All of life shares the common life cycle of birth, growth, harvest, and rest. In our work, this cycle might be training $\longrightarrow$ experience $\longrightarrow$ expertise $\longrightarrow$ acceptance or respect. In our relationships, it might be attraction $\longrightarrow$ growth of love $\longrightarrow$ communication $\longrightarrow$ harmony or comfort. In our individual lives, there is the overall cycle from childhood and adolescence (birth) $\longrightarrow$ early adulthood (growth) $\longrightarrow$ middle age (harvest) $\longrightarrow$ older age (rest).[2]

Yin-yang is a tool and a toy which we can use to help us harmonize our individual lives with the changes in Nature. In a sense, we are always in harmony with Nature, for we ARE Nature. But sometimes we feel as though we are being jerked around, as though our lives are full of fairly continuous abrupt changes. As we use yin-yang to understand the process of change—and first just to see and accept the fact of change—we find life flowing more smoothly. The journey through life is rather like driving a car. If we steer by jerking the wheel first way to the right, then

---

[1] *Nei Ching*, from section 25.

[2] In different cultures, different balances of yin and yang exist in general for each different age; for example, in the later years of life might be times of more rest than earlier periods, but still times of activity and positive contribution to the society.

way to the left, the car may stay on the road —but we are working pretty hard to keep it there. If we understand how the steering wheel works, and turn it just slightly to the right, and slightly to the left, the same or better effects are achieved more smoothly and the ride is more pleasant and joyous.

Ki, the Vital Life Force

Ki is an energy more primal than that of the endocrine, nervous, or circulatory systems. The classics say that "blood follows ki"—this means that even so fundamental a life support system as the blood and vascular system is dependent upon and derives its well-being from the state of the ki. Ki is an energy finer than that of electricity or electromagnetic energy. It is, really, the basic energy of life, of the Tao. The determination of a person's current ki state and of practices and techniques to balance and replenish that ki state are basic to any traditional oriental therapies or health arts.

Though all ki is basically the same vital energy, every animal and plant has its own form of ki just as every species has its own forms of physical nourishment. When living beings take in food, their bodies break down the chemically complex food materials so that the nutrients present—carbohydrates, fats, protein, vitamins, mineral, and water— can be used in the thousands of internal chemical reactions that maintain life. In a similar way, living beings absorb the ki of heaven (through the breath) and the ki of earth (through food), then combine these to form that being's own "true ki" or life energy.

The vital energy, or ki, of the body flows both externally (below the surface of the skin) and internally (within the deeper tissues and organs) along definite, orderly pathways throughout the body. These pathways, found in all living creatures, are called "meridians"

and "channels." Their routes have been traced and diagramed since ancient times and also using modern scientific research methods. The classics say that health and happiness abound when the ki flows freely through these pathways in a steady and orderly way, being neither too active (yang) nor too passive (yin). The ki then vitalizes all the cells, tissues, organs, and systems of the body, and integrates them in function.

Acu-points are, traditionally speaking, points where the ki flow comes to the surface of the body. Scientifically speaking, these points (tsubo) are essentially points of high electrical conductivity or, conversely, low electrical resistance. They act somewhat like amplifiers, passing the ki along from one point to another. The meridians and the channels are the transmission lines along which the ki flows. These points and lines are not visible to the eye, but it is possible, under some circumstances, to feel the ki flowing through them.

In meditation or meditation-in-action (such as T'ai Chi Chu'an, or the external exercises of Taoist yoga) one can actually become aware of one's ki. Beyond that, one can feel its flow through the body and eventually even map part or all of its routes. This is how the meridians and channels of acupuncture and acupressure were originally discovered, and even today this spontaneous and intuitive method of discovery is not uncommon. Jiro Murai, the master who transmitted the ancient acupressure technique of Jin Shin to the present, experienced the body's ki flow in just this way, as have recluses and mystics through the ages.

During research in Japan, it was explained that Jiro Murai had ruined his health with excessive living and by the time he was in his early twenties had become dangerously ill. His father and uncle were doctors, but neither they nor anyone else could help him. Always an independent person, Jiro Murai said, "At least I can choose the way I wish to die." He insisted upon being carried up to the top of the mountains where he would starve to death.

In the mountains, Jiro Murai recalled the strange energy flows throughout the human body which were a part of the folk understanding of early times. He remembered the hand positions shown in statues of Buddha—which are found everywhere in the Japanese countryside and cities—and he experimented with these simple meditation postures while waiting for his death.

After a few days, he felt very hot. He began to feel "rivers of fire" running through his body. Using the hand positions, he was able to feel his flows of energy, or "meridians" and "channels," and even to map them. (His later drawings of the energy flows he had felt are very similar to the acupuncture charts handed down since ancient times.) Fasting had made Jiro Murai extremely sensitive to and aware of these energies; soon he was able to control them.

When this was over, Jiro Murai was completely well. He fell to his knees in gratitude and vowed to heaven that he would look into these ancient wisdoms and bring them back to mankind. He donated his findings to one of the oldest shrines in Japan, the Ise Shrine near Osaka. From then on, he traveled through Japan developing methods of balancing the ki so as to help others. To those who would listen, he taught simple ways of helping control one's own ki through acupressure and through meditation.

At this time, Japan as a whole was turning away from its traditional culture and eagerly embracing the modern western ways. The world as a whole was turning away from the wisdom of the ancients, and eagerly embracing the knowledge of modern science and technology. Now, nearly half a century later, we are seeing that the new world has need of the old; the West has need of the East; the

scientific method has need of the intuitive vision. For the few who maintained and developed the ancient wisdoms, and for their students who transmitted these to the present, we who follow must be deeply grateful. The gifts are not without the givers.

Jin Shin Do acupressure, which derives from the discoveries of Jiro Murai and of other masters, is an inherently meditative technique. It encourages a state of relaxation similar to that experienced in deep meditation—a state in which one can experience one's ki and often, if sufficiently relaxed and receptive, even feel it "streaming" or "flowing" through the body. At the end of a Jin Shin Do acupressure treatment, recipients usually feel a general sensation of ki flow that takes them out of the material realm and into a different realm of consciousness. We might call this an "alpha-wave" state; it can also be experienced during "hara breathing" or other forms of meditation—and indeed in any truly creative experience, be it music, art, communication, carpentry, or whatever.

Some recipients of Jin Shin Do acupressure treatments are sensitive enough to very clearly describe parts of the ki flow that they are experiencing. In hearing these descriptions, as well as in my own experiences, I have been amazed at their coincidence with the ancient energy maps. I have also been continuously amazed at the ease with which either receiving or doing a Jin Shin treatment can transport almost anyone to a different plane of being—where things seem suddenly clearer, brighter, and more easily flowing.

Acupuncture and acupressure theory and technique arose from such direct and indirect experience of the ki, or vital energy, more than 5000 years ago. Today, the existence of ki is a basic premise of these arts. However, we can ourselves both experience and even scientifically research this basic premise.

As early as 1940, Russian scientists, led by

Semyon and Valentina Kirlian, had developed techniques for making images of this energy as seen in human beings and in other life forms. Basically, they used photography with high frequency electrical fields which caused objects to radiate an energy field, appearing as lines and points of colored light, onto photo paper. This "Kirlian photography" provided the first, now fairly well-known, scientific evidence of the existence of the "life energy" (ki) which had been the basis of oriental therapies and health practices for thousands of years.

Many researchers in the West have now experimented with Kirlian photography—notably Moss and Johnson at the University of California, Los Angeles.[1] The Kirlian photographs show both external and internal patterns of living objects; typical effects are "fields" surrounding the objects (or subjects) photographed. Kirlian photographs of leaves plucked from plants show smaller and smaller fields as the leaves turn brown and die. Kirlian photographs of the human fingertips show full and balanced oval fields in healthy persons; smaller and more chaotic fields in distraught or imbalanced persons. Thus the "fields" seem to correlate with the health or dis-ease of a living organism. Many researchers feel that they are visual representations of a "bioenergy"—the ancient "ki flow."

Kirlian photography is but one of a growing number of ways in which modern western and eastern scientists have been experimenting with and attempting to understand or verify the concept of ki. Although much of this research has been very recent, earlier in this century the great psychologist Wilhelm Reich had already discovered this life energy. Calling it "orgone energy," he scientifically experimented with and observed it, learning in detail the relationship between physical tensions or armoring (blocking the flow of this basic life energy) and mental or emotional difficulties.

Jin Shin Do: Ki Release and Redirection

The great ancient religions and philosophies of all cultures included an understanding of the universal life force, ki. This was fundamental to ancient Taoism. As John Blofeld, an amazing journeyer with the ability to both absorb and transmit, writes: "Taoist painting and poetry can be seen to reflect a direct perception and conscious experience of nature's functioning, which has little in common with the analytical approach of geologists, botanists and other exponents of the natural sciences. The Taoists, like Wordsworth, perceived that the universe is a living organism, that its groves and streams are interfused with mysterious spirit, its rocks and mountains endowed with life-force."[2] Not only man, but all of nature participates in the flow of universal energy—ki.

Now, we in the West are beginning to see this life force in the form of Kirlian photographs, record its activities in scientific experiments of many types, and feel it ourselves in meditation and in health arts. We have finally broken past our skepticism and are in a position to begin using Lao Tzu's three—yin-yang, and ki.

Through the meridians or ki pathways, the surrounding energies of the universe

[1]Some pertinent research reports: "Photographic Evidence of Healing Energy on Plants and People," Thelma Moss, Kendall Johnson, Marshall Barshay, and Jack Gray, Dimensions of Healing Symposium, University Extension, UCIA, 1972;

"Visual Evidence of Bioenergetic Interactions Between People?," Thelma Moss, John Hubacher, and Frances Saba, UCLA Neuropsychiatric Institute, Center for the Health Sciences; presented at the American Psychiatric Association, May, 1974.

[2]The Secret and the Sublime: Taoist Mysteries and Magic, by John Blofeld, Dutton, New York, 1973, page 114.

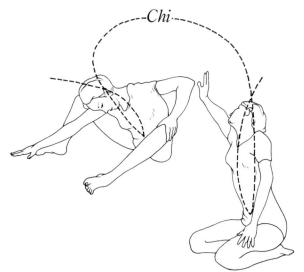

communicate with man. Ki flows through the meridians of our energy bodies just as food and liquid flow through the digestive and assimilative systems of our material bodies. The ki flow through the meridians is our "energy body."

Ki within our bodies is ki that we have taken in from the universe. It is ki that other beings (plants, animals, men, and other living creatures) have previously used and expelled. Thus each person is actually a purification or toxification unit for this energy. If we each gradually purify the ki within our own bodies and progressively clear our own energy channels, we are both participating more fully in the universal vital energy ourselves and, by giving off clearer ki, enabling other beings to do so as well. We are, by helping ourselves and our friends, making an actual change in the entire scheme of the ten thousand things.

Just as each thought we send out carries its own vibration and sets into action physical and emotional cause-and-effect changes, so the ki we expel goes on to other beings and motivates them in higher or lower ways. This is one reason why the mere presence of a happy person evokes feelings of peace, calm, and joy, while the mere presence of an unhappy person can evoke feelings of anxiety, irritation, or depression. Energy does not disappear, nor is it dissipated. It is merely transformed, transmuted, and transmitted.

The ancient health practices of Jin Shin Do are designed to strengthen our absorption of the life energy, and to balance and direct its flow through our body, so that it follows its proper course. When tension develops and the bodily ki flows stagnate or deviate, the accompanying physical malfunctioning can cause dis-ease to occur in the body. When we are blocked, we perceive the Tao, the one, the two (yin and yang), and the three (yin-yang and ki) as though through a foggy glass. We become almost totally preoccupied with and worried about the ten thousand things—the material world. Losing contact with Tao (Nature, or God), we alienate ourselves from the divine healing energies.

Jin Shin Do acupressure treatments are based on the release of points or body areas at which tension, blockage, and stagnation of the ki flow usually occur. In its release techniques, Jin Shin Do uses the pathways through which the body regulates and balances its ki flow. Thus Jin Shin Do treatments help the body to regain its physical, emotional, mental, spiritual, and energic balance. From this balance between the yin (passivity) and the yang (activity) flow thoughts, feelings, and actions through which the individual can effect wider and wider spheres of consciousness.

If one does not aim at balancing the ki when practicing oriental health arts, then one continues to work superficially. Ki is the most primal energy, the basic energy of life. Ki manifests. Matter—the body, a tree, a house, the earth—is, in oriental terms, "frozen ki" (or ki that is moving at a slower rate of vibration). To effect the most fundamental change, we must release and balance the ki. We may also need to directly work on transforming the physical, emotional, and mental conditions which influence the ki state, but even these can also be transmuted through control of the ki. This basic understanding made all oriental therapies and health arts preventative rather than symptomatic in nature.

3. KNOWING OURSELVES

"He who knows others is wise;
He who knows himself is enlightened."[1]

The Yin and Yang of Human Expectations

Everything changes from yin to yang to yin to yang continuously. This perception of cyclic (and spirallic) change can improve the quality of our individual lives immensely, for it can liberate us from the tunnel vision which causes so much of our unhappiness. We constantly get ourselves either into situations which we regard as "bad" and fear will continue for a long time, or else into situations which we regard as "good" and fear won't continue forever. We might call the former a "punishment syndrome" and the latter a "pleasure syndrome." Both are equally destructive to our happiness and self-development, and both derive from basic personal insecurity, fixation on "good" and "bad," and lack of understanding of or faith in the order of universal change.

The yin-yang principle teaches us that nothing continues forever, and nothing is inherently good or bad. "Good" and "bad" is a dualism having to do with the relationship of events to human goals and desires, and is not a quality inherent in the nature of things. Furthermore, our conception of even our own lives, let alone the life of the Universe, is too limited for us to truly judge what is really good and what is really bad. Many times we reject, rebel against, complain about, or are distressed because of events which in retrospect were necessary to our growth, accomplishments, understanding, or general happiness.

Throughout oriental philosophy, in every culture, we find both creation and destruction—building up and breaking down—portrayed together, as the two hands of God. Thus, even Tara (Kuan Yin, embodiment of compassion energy), though she usually appears as a serene, beautiful, angelic goddess, also has her fierce, devilish form. To label one or the other as "good" or "bad" would have amazed the ancients, for it is synonymous to rejecting half of existence rather than embracing the Tao—All that is. The point is that while we can use the "good-bad" dualism, we do not need to label everything with it. If we chronically do so, we tend to get into tunnel visions, wherein we see only the hoped-for "good" or dreaded "bad"—cutting ourselves off from a whole spectrum of perceptions and in effect being used by our own ideas of good and bad.

How can we get out of our tunnel visions? How can we transform the punishment and pleasure syndromes? The dynamic yin-yang principle is an ancient tool for erasing tunnels by revealing a different and more inclusive perspective of life.

If we are in a difficult or "bad" situation, and we fear it will continue for a long time, then what we must do is firstly see the prob-

---

[1] *Tao Teh Ching*, from Chapter XXVIII.

lem for what it is and secondly see how it may change or be transmuted. For example, our problem may be that we are in a professional or personal situation which we do not like. We feel that we are stagnating and going nowhere, or even regressing. There is a Japanese phrase describing this feeling: "hai-iro no seikatsu"—literally, life has the color and taste of ashes. Though we can interpret this situation as "bad," in reality it is only yin— too passive and therefore stagnant. Yin at its extreme necessarily and naturally changes to yang: we may be promoted or recognized; we may discover a new or deeper professional or personal interest; or we may find ourselves being propelled even without our conscious volition out of the situation.

On the other hand, perhaps we have just been promoted into a situation we have wanted for a long time, or have just found a new and deep love. The pleasure syndrome arises: "This is so good, it can't last!" From that, the correlate: "This is so good, I've got to hold onto it!" By our fears and worries, we may in fact create fears or vibrations which end the promotion or alienate the loved one. By our clinging to excitement and pleasure, we can also be borne up on an almost hysterical balloon of jubilation which, being an extreme, can easily be popped. If we discover difficult aspects of the situation—the greater work demands of our new profession or position, or the personal difficulties of our loved one—or are rejected after being initially accepted, then we are crushed. We must learn to accept and enjoy happiness as our birthright and difficulties as our teachers, and then we will not need to cling so desperately to the peaks of the waves.

The goal of the oriental seeker was not to embrace the good and reject the bad, but to embrace all phenomena and non-phenomena, irrespective of their relative merits, and to live in harmony with Nature's subtle but great Truth of Change. Yin changes into

yang, yang changes into yin; the spiral of change is continuous. If we can grow to really incorporate that principle into our lives, we can flow much more smoothly and joyfully with life's changes.

Alan Watts, who probably did more than any other philosopher introduced the West to the Taoist Way, related an old story exemplifying this Way: A farmer had only one horse. One day, his horse ran away. "That evening the neighbors gathered to commiserate with him since this was such bad luck. He said, 'May be.' The next day the horse returned, but brought with it six wild horses, and the neighbors came exclaiming at his good fortune. He said, 'May be.' And then, the following day, his son tried to saddle and ride one of the wild horses, was thrown, and broke his leg. Again the neighbors came to offer their sympathy for the misfortune. He said, 'May be.' The day after that, conscription officers came to the village to seize young men for the army, but because of the broken leg the farmer's son was rejected. When the neighbors came in to say how fortunately everything had turned out, he said, 'May be.' "[1] The authors comment: "The yin-yang view of the world is serenely cyclic."[1]

Summer changes into winter, and winter into summer, continuously. The sun rises and sets, the moon waxes and wanes. The tide ebbs and recedes. Leaves change from green to brown, and the sky from light to dark. We are in no way separate from nature. And we are not only a part of nature; we are nature too. Our lives also flow in harmony with the cosmic changes. The expression of this is the purpose of the yin-yang principle. The experience of this is the aim of all traditional oriental health arts.

To attach our happiness to the attainment

[1]Tao: The Watercourse Way, by Alan Watts, with Al Chung-Liang Huang, Pantheon Books, Random House, New York, 1975, page 31.

of certain goals or desires, and not to also be open to what the flow of life's changes brings, is to be happy during very limited periods of time. Unless our happiness is in the process of growth, the experience of unfolding awareness, all the changes of the spiral, and not just in attainment of specific material or ego-bolstering goals, we deny ourselves happiness throughout about 350 degrees of each revolution!

KARMA IS FOR GROWING

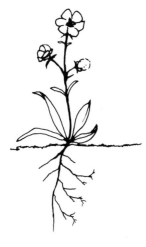

The soil is to the flower's growth what our karma (life events and difficulties) is to our growth. The soil both provides the nutrients the flower needs for growth, and at the same time is a barrier against which the tender young plant must push until it reaches the light of the sun.

We want life to be as happy as possible. But real happiness lies only in ultimate enlightenment—not in becoming what we think we should be, not in becoming what others think we should be, but rather in becoming ourselves, realizing our Tao-nature, uncovering or freeing our inner Spirit (Shin).

That progressive clarity and freedom don't happen easily. Neither does the young sprout easily push its way through the soil which surrounds and nurtures it. Difficulties, problems, dilemmas are to us what the soil is to the plant: both barriers and also nourishment. They nurture our growth by teaching us, by making us expand our limits. If we can learn to enjoy and appreciate both front and back, all of our karma, then we can grow towards the spiritual sun. That sun, the light of the Tao, is as necessary to our real aliveness as the earthly sun is to the flower.

The Yin and Yang of Our Physical Conditions

We have explored the yin-yang philosophy in some depth in order to: 1) see and understand the nature of change more clearly, 2) learn to use this ancient tool for self-growth, and 3) be able to balance the physical condition through the use of ancient oriental health arts. As we now turn to this third aspect of yin-yang study, we will find that what we have learned from observing the macrocosm—Nature—will facilitate our understanding of the microcosm—the human condition. What we have learned from considering the mind—the emotional and spiritual as well as intellectual natures—will apply to the body—the physical condition.

First, what is a yin physical condition, and what is a yang physical condition? This is a question which we could explore in great detail, but the basic outline of its answer can be seen quite easily. Yin is passive; yang is active. Therefore, a person who is usually more passive physically will generally be in a more yin condition. A person who is usually more active physically will generally be in a more yang condition. Using the yin-yang principle to look at specific body states, cramped muscles would be yang and flaccid muscles yin; hypertension (high blood pressure) would be yang and hypotension yin; insomnia would be yang and general drowsiness yin; being "hyped up" would be yang and being generally fatigued would be yin. (It is to be noted that these are really extremes of yin and yang.) Heat is yang; coolness is yin. Therefore, fevers would generally be yang and chills would be yin. (Since these are extreme conditions, one can turn into the other.) If the feet and hands are usually cold, or if the person is very sensitive to cold, the condition would be more yin. If the hands are generally too warm, the face flushed, or the body feeling warm in general, the condition is more yang. Difficult or forced breathing would be yang; weak or shallow breathing would be yin.

Determining the basic yin-yang condition is indispensable to proper Jin Shin Do acupressure technique. It involves observing many different aspects of the body-mind condition —those mentioned above, the pulse, and the physiognomy, for example. It is also an intuitive understanding. If a person walks into a room briskly and acts energetically and decisively, or even tends to pace the room restlessly, and talks in a clear and strong voice, we feel that person to be in a more yang condition. If, on the other hand, someone walks into a room slowly, has a drooping posture, tends to be lethargic or lazy, and talks very softly or haltingly, we feel that person to be in a more yin condition.

The person in a more yang condition may have more or deeper muscular tension. He or she has plenty of energy, or ki, but may become fatigued or less effective in action because the ki is blocked up in various places of tension and therefore not fully available for use. The person in a more yin condition may have less or less extensive muscular tension, and he or she is generally weaker physically. This person may be deficient in energy, or ki, and may need to nourish and replenish it (as through dietary and life-style changes) in addition to releasing the muscular blocks and balancing the energy condition.

The acupressure technique will vary accordingly. A firmer pressure (though not an excessive one) can be used with the more yang person, and more attention can be given to muscular release. A gentler pressure must be used with the more yin person, and more attention must be given to channeling the ki or energy (which will be discussed in the next chapter). The more yang person can benefit from exercise and breathing techniques directed towards releasing areas of muscular tension. The more yin person should learn exercise and breathing techniques for increasing the ki, and for gradually developing muscular strength as well.

As we begin to use yin and yang to consider physical conditions, two important aspects of yin-yang philosophy must be remembered. Firstly, yin and yang are both positive in that they are both vital and necessary forces of life. Yin is often defined as negative ($-$) and yang as positive ($+$), but these should not be taken in any way to mean that yin is "bad" and yang is "good." Positive and negative are used in the sense of being complimentary and relative opposites, as in chemistry. To be active and energetic is desirable, but to be quiet and relaxed is also desirable! What is needed is to become balanced, to embrace both the yin and the yang, and to harmonize their cyclic interaction.

Becoming balanced, embracing both the yang and the yin—what do these mean? The oriental ideal of physical balance is to be yang on the inside and yin on the outside—to have strong internal organs and metabolism, but to have flexible muscles and tendons.

Many times, with the pressures of modern life and the conditions of modern life styles, we have become just the opposite—weak internally and tense or rigid externally.

The Taoist ideal of psychological balance is to embrace both the female and male sides of our natures—to be both receptive and active according to circumstance. Though yin is classified as female (and vice versa), and yang as male, nothing is totally yin or totally yang. Which is to say, we are all in a sense androgynous. Development of both sides of our being is necessary for our completion as women, as men, as people. The most masculine male is not only strong and active, but also gentle and receptive. The most feminine female is not only gentle and receptive, but also strong and active. "Strong and active" means assertive, and not aggressive (which is an extreme). "Gentle and receptive" means accepting, and not dependent (which is an extreme).

We can use the yin-yang principle to help create a dynamic balance of yin and yang in our physical conditions and in our life-styles. In body-mind work, this yin-yang balance has several aspects. These include balance of the physical structure, the emotional state, the intellectual processes, the spiritual being, and the energic being. Balancing the latter, the vital energy or ki, as well as opening and centering Shin, the Spirit, are the most fundamental. While the balance of the ki and the condition of Shin are influenced by all the other aspects of the being, to a large degree (according to the ancient oriental wisdom) it is the state of the ki and of Shin which governs the body and mind. The yin-yang balance of the ki, which can be controlled by the Spirit, creates the bodily harmony or disharmony.

The second aspect of the yin-yang philosophy which must be remembered when we consider the yin and yang of physical conditions is that yin and yang are relative. They are opposite but complementary aspects of the One. Without yin, yang cannot exist; without yang, yin cannot exist. Dark and light, night and day, earth and heaven, front and back—all exist only by virtue of each other and in relation to each other. "Heaviness is the basis of lightness; calmness is the controlling power of hastiness."[1] Things are yin or yang only in relation to other things.

Therefore, we really should not say "earth is yin" and "heaven is yang." Earth is yin in relation to heaven; heaven is yang in relation to earth. Earth is also yin in relation to the sun, which is very much warmer than the earth. But earth is yang in relation to the moon, which is cooler and contains less life energy than the earth. So when we say "earth is yin and heaven is yang," we must remember that this is so only within that comparison.

Another part of this relativity is that nothing, except the "Yin" and "Yang" principles themselves, is entirely yin or entirely yang. In the yin-yang symbol, we see a little circle of yin (black) in the yang (white) part, and a little circle of yang (white) in the yin (black) part. This is a symbolic representation of the fact that all things contain both yin and yang, though in varying proportions.

Therefore, whenever we refer to another person from the viewpoint of yin and yang, or look at ourselves and our own lives from this point of view, we must remember the relativity of this principle as well as its dynamic nature. We must remember that yin and yang are not absolutes, but are constantly-changing and relative conditions. That is why, in referring to a person, oriental therapists usually follow the word "yin" or "yang" with some word such as "sei," which means condition. To quote a primary philosopher of oriental therapeutics, George Ohsawa:

---

[1] *Tao Teh Ching*, from Chapter XXVI.

"In other words, to say 'He is yin' is not really accurate; it means he is absolutely and forever yin, Yin itself, but one is really only presently manifesting Yin or Yang (actually both, of course). So it would be more accurate to say 'He is yin-sei.' (Sei means character, quality, state, condition, nature, etc.) Everything is made by Yin and Yang, never equal to Yin or Yang. (Or both: as part of the whole, we can never equal it.)"[1]

Even some oriental doctors analyze a person as "yin" or "yang" and then tell him how to behave within that context. This is to ignore the basic truth of eternal change, which means that anything can and does change. We can change our condition; we can change our lives; we can change almost everything, for everything changes. Sometimes conditions which are further progressed in either direction are actually easier to change. The person who experiences many difficulties often comes to see himself more clearly and more deeply desires to change. The one who has only very minor complaints will perhaps not reflect so deeply or have so strong a desire to change until his or her situation becomes more acute. Thus there is an old oriental saying, "He who has one disease, or one problem, is fortunate."

Jin Shin Do is built on the foundation of yin-yang thinking. Thus it is a philosophy and technique of change, of change not in a violent or chaotic way, but rather in a naturally smooth, orderly, and simple way. The possibilities for personal change are limited primarily by our own understanding of and desire for change.

The art of using yin and yang in our lives is to realize that all things consist of both. Even if one overwhelmingly dominates the other, there is always at least the seed of the other hidden within its depths—ready to sprout, grow, and eventually become an equally potent force.

"Please bear in mind that the power of Heaven is great and that it can change ill luck for the better. Outside of all living creation and within the Universe are transformations brought about by Heaven and Earth and by the interrelation of Yin and Yang."[2]

Where Have We Come From?

We can use the ancient tool of "physiognomy"—study of the face—to get a glimpse of our "original constitution"—our condition of yin-yang balance at birth. This original constitution is the foundation of our physical and mental condition throughout life. Though the possible changes for each individual are infinite, the ease or difficulty of changing is conditioned by this original constitution.

What determines our original constitution? A multitude of natural forces including the genetic inheritance of our parents, the location and season of our birth, the dietary and living habits of our mother, and the relationship of our planet to other celestial bodies. All of these and many other influences play a role in determining our condition at birth.

If we were active babies, demanding attention and being very alert and curious, our original constitution was probably "yang" —the yang forces were dominant. If our disposition was more passive, if we were quiet and easy to take care of, our original constitution was probably more "yin"—the yin forces were dominant. Neither of these

---

[1] *Four Hours to Basic Japanese*, by George Ohsawa, George Ohsawa Macrobiotic Foundation.
[2] *Nei Ching*, from section 17.

conditions are in themselves good or bad; however, extremes of either condition can cause their respective problems.

According to the ancients, the body structure also tells the story of our original constitution. A thin-boned or tall structure is usually more yin; a thick-boned or short structure is usually more yang. The bone structure of the face is an especially accurate record. Though there are many signs which could be observed, just the basic shape of the face tells a great deal.

Get out a mirror and see if you can discover which of these six basic facial shapes is yours:

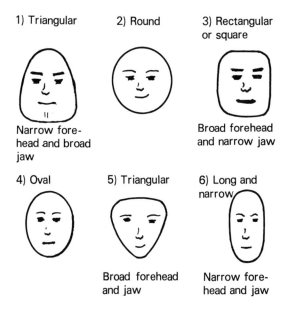

1) Triangular

Narrow forehead and broad jaw

2) Round

3) Rectangular or square

Broad forehead and narrow jaw

4) Oval

5) Triangular

Broad forehead and jaw

6) Long and narrow

Narrow forehead and jaw

The first shape is a sign of a very yang original constitution. This type of person is generally physically strong and also strong-willed. Type two is also yang and has similar tendencies depending on the breadth of the jaw. Type three is the most yang, tending to be the most assertive personality and tending to have highly-developed practical thinking skills. These persons may wish to become more open to the emotional and intuitive sides of their natures.

Type four is evidence of a balanced original constitution, with neither yang nor yin forces being dominant. People of this type may tend to be more flexible in life-style and attitude than individuals of either yang or yin original constitution. They will more frequently have developed both the physical or practical and the intellectual or artistic sides of their natures, to some degree. These persons may tend to have fewer difficulties, and may tend to seek difficulties (consciously or unconsciously) to develop themselves and grow in understanding.

Persons with facial type five are generally of a more yin original constitution. They may not be as strong physically as the first four types, and may tend to be more cerebral in their orientation. Often these persons are the most intellectual, artistic, or mystical, relying for survival upon their innate powers of thinking and intuition rather than upon their physical strength (which of course they may develop). The sixth type is the most yin in original constitution, sharing the characteristics of type five, but perhaps more strongly needing to develop physical strength and will.

Of course, there are an infinite number of faces in this world, and so there are an infinite number of face shapes. If you can look closely and objectively, you can see which of these six basic shapes yours most closely resembles, and then see how strongly you might share the characteristic tendencies.

There are a number of other signs in the face that can give clear insight into the original constitution. A few of the most easily observed are:

A protruding chin or a cleft in the chin are further signs of yang dominance; while a receding chin is a further sign of yin dominance.

Long, well-shaped earlobes are a sign of strong innate vitality, or pre-natal ki.

Strong, clear-cut features in general are signs of yang dominance.

Who Have We Become?

As we develop, the experiences and forces of life—and our reaction to them—produce an ever-evolving, ever new self. Our "acquired constitution"—our here-and-now condition of yin-yang balance or imbalance—is thus constantly changing and capable of being changed. This acquired constitution may closely reflect our original constitution, or it may show a great change from our condition at birth.

This acquired constitution is seen in the soft tissues of the body, rather than in the bony structure, for the former are more easily influenced by our life-style and environment. Our acquired constitution is that which we have become, that which we have made of ourselves.

In searching our physiognomy for this acquired constitution, we may come across aspects of our condition which we wish to change, as well as aspects which we are happy to see. It is very important that we learn to greet both "good" and "bad" discoveries with interest and joy, for it is only through self-awareness that lasting change can come. We can learn to say "Hey, how about that! There's something else to work on!" with the amazement and joy of a child learning about life.

For the process of self-discovery and self-growth is itself fun—joy does not lie only in end results. The sooner we let go of the illusion that we are now or soon will (or must) be perfect, the more joyous and full of growth our lives will be. What replaces perfection as a goal? Openness to continual growth—which is always beautiful, as is the health and well-being which accompany increasing awareness. Our physiognomy is really a personal mandala which can guide our self-reflection and meditation in this process.

"Thinking that one knows when one does not know is sickness. Only when one becomes sick of this sickness can one be free from sickness."

There are dozens of signs in the face indicating our acquired constitutions. However, it is unnecessary to go into all these details in order to see our basic present yin-yang condition. Perhaps the first place to look is the eyes, for it is said "the eyes reflect Shin." A strong Shin, or Spirit, is reflected in shining, clear, animated eyes, while a weak Spirit is reflected in lackluster, cloudy, or dull eyes.

The position of the colored part of the eyes relative to the whites reveals the condition of the overall body energy. If the body is in a balanced state, the eye will be centered as in Figure 1 below. If the white of the eye is visible below the iris (Figure 2), the body is in a yin energy state. In this case, there is not enough energy to nourish and sustain the body, and the person may be accident-prone and easily depressed. The larger the white area under the eye, the more severe and chronic the condition may be. This yin *sanpaku* condition is frequently seen in photographs of persons who have committed suicide (though it does not necessarily mean a tendency to that action). Slight and temporary conditions of yin sanpaku may result from fatigue.

Figure 1   **Figure 2**   **Figure 3**

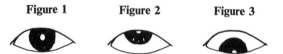

In the opposite instance, called yang sanpaku, the whites of the eye are visible above the iris (Figure 3). This may indicate an excess of energy—or, rather, an excess of energy that is not being used, since there is almost no limit to the amount of ki that one can store and use. The person may be hyperactive and may tend to be irritable. In severe cases, this condition may indicate anger or a lack of control, and the person may tend to be dangerous to others. A temporary yang sanpaku condition may occur when a person is very excited or eager about something he or she is discussing.

The area directly under the lower eyelid reflects the condition of the "ki of generative force," the reserve energy stored in the kidneys and *hara* (vital center in the lower abdomen). If this area is dark, swollen, lined, or bumpy, it indicates a lack of this reserve energy and therefore a tendency to physical or emotional fatigue. Before there can be reserve energy, there must be sufficient ki for all the body's normal maintenance functions. Therefore, general body strengthening and release is indicated first, including sufficient rest and nourishment as well as overall energy release and balancing. Hara breathing (see next chapter) can be used to increase and store body energy, but emotional causes—fear and paranoia—must also be considered.

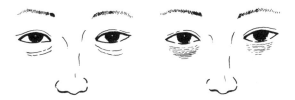

Swollen Area Under Eyes   Dark Area Under Eyes

Because the pace of modern life is so rapid, with so many different pressures and attractions, and because our culture has not generally emphasized or even taught methods of accumulating and storing energy, some degree of this condition is very common. It can be seen even in very small children. As we import and practice oriental methods of self-cultivation, in addition to using historical and newly-discovered western methods, perhaps a balance to our western trends of productivity and constant animation will be established.

A pair of furrows between the eyebrows can indicate toxicity of the liver, or can be a sign of repressed frustration and anger. The person may "explode" if the internal tension becomes extreme. In addition to releasing tension, the condition can also be improved by dealing with the sources of the anger and frustration and by using anger energy in physical activity and in work directed towards accomplishment of a dream.

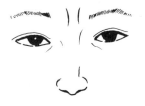

Furrows Between Eyebrows

The current yin-yang condition can also be seen in the mouth. If the teeth are clenched tight, the lips are drawn in, and there is tension in the jaw muscles, the person's condition is too yang. The digestive system may also be contracted and tense, and there may be physical or mental constipation. If the lips are expanded, and especially if the jaw muscles are flaccid and the mouth tends to hang open, the condition is too yin. The digestive system may be expanded and weak, and the person may suffer from a resultant lack of energy. There may be diarrhoea, or there may be "yin constipation" (eliminatory problems resulting from a lack of peristaltic action rather than from tension as in "yang constipation").

Pulse reading is also a very important means of determining both general and also very specific conditions of current yin-yang balance or imbalance. Though pulse reading cannot be learned from a book, the reader can at least begin to explore the basics of this amazing oriental art. There are three pulse positions on each hand (see illustration). The middle (second) position is located on the radial artery horizontal to the styloid process or protrusion at the end of the radius bone of the forearm extending from the (elbow to the thumb). The first and third positions are located just above and below this middle one. In taking the pulses on yourself or on others, your index finger should palpate the first pulse position, your middle finger the second, and your ring finger the third.

There are two depths—"superficial" and "deep"—at each pulse position. But to feel the general yin-yang condition, it is sufficient at first to just apply moderate pressure to all three positions on each hand. If the pulse feels strong and full, or even pounding like waves in the ocean, the condition is probably yang. If the pulse feels weak and delicate, or is difficult to feel, the condition is probably yin.

In determining both your original constitution and your acquired condition, all of these and other conditions must be considered together. Usually we find that we have some yin indications, some yang, and some balanced. To see the general tendencies, it may be helpful to make a check-list. Take a piece of paper and head one column "original constitution" and the other "acquired condition." List all the relevant factors under each, and see if you can discover where you have come from and who you have become.

Left

Right

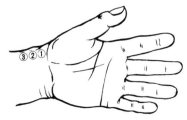 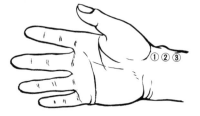

4. MAGIC IN YOUR FINGERTIPS:
The Inner Art of Channeling Ki

A great ocean of ki surrounds and envelops us. As we choose, we are either rocks against which the waves of universal energy crash and disperse, or else sponges absorbing its magical, life-nourishing waters. It is this great ocean of universal energy that we must learn to contact, absorb, and channel, if our acupressure treatments are to be the truly magical ways to more radiant health that they can be.

In acupuncture, needles are used to achieve "teh chi"—tapping of the chi, or ki—so that energy can be dispersed from an area if it is in excess or drawn to the area if the ki is deficient there. Needles can be, in the hands of skilled and moderately enlightened practitioners, very wonderful tools. But there is no stronger conductor of ki in the world than the human hand. In order to channel the universal energy through our hands, we must ourselves achieve "teh chi," tapping the great ocean of ki.

Every person has some amount of ki circulating in his or her own body, and concentrated in the various body centers. Unless a simple meditative process is used to tap the Big Ki, when we first use our hands in treatments to help others we may instead draw on our own Little (or bodily) Ki. That is why, after attempting palm healing or other "laying on of hands" techniques on their own,

sometimes people report feeling very fatigued or even ill after working on someone else. This draining of the treater's energy can be especially strong when he or she is working on a loved one, someone for whom there is a great deal of care and concern.

This is not necessary. Every person has the ability to give not just of his or her own bodily ki, but to tap and channel from the great ocean of vital energy that is all around us. If this ability is developed and used, even beginners feel invigorated after working on someone else. In the process, they have increased their own absorption and internal channeling of ki, as well as that of their friend or family member.

Some people intuitively know how to channel energy, and perhaps do so spontaneously and naturally that they may not even be aware of the process. But, like most gifts, the ability to channel and balance ki can be developed by almost anyone. If you have compassion for and sincerely desire to help others, you can learn to give very effective Jin Shin Do treatments—and to yourself reach higher levels of freedom, clarity, well-being, and happiness in the process.

An analogy is the gift of music and the ability to sing. In the West, many people have been inculcated with the idea that music is a special faculty given by the gods, as it were,

42

to a few. In questioning people who "just can't carry a tune" or cannot play any sort of musical instrument, it will usually be found that they either were not encouraged musically as children, or were actually discouraged by actions or attitudes of parents and peers (which include unpleasant or forced introductions to music). On the other hand, in a society in which people are expected to be musical, they are musical. In Japan, for instance, it is almost a part of the folklore that "every Japanese can sing." And so they can! Even today, in clubs throughout Japan, there will often be a professional musician (maybe doubling as a waiter), but perhaps half the audience will also take a turn singing —and will sing as well as the professional.

Like the tradition that "everyone can sing," in the Orient traditionally almost everyone could treat with his or her hands. Most people knew at least a few strong points, and a simple technique of holding these points, in order to help themselves, their families, and their friends. Perhaps the day is not so far off when this will also be true in the West. In order for that day to dawn, we must rediscover the magic that is in our fingertips—the power of the energy which we can channel through our hands.

Learning how to channel ki by means of simple meditative practices—and by creative visualization—is important in the practice of Jin Shin Do. With this ability, one is an artist; without it, one is only a mechanic— though perhaps a good one. One can begin as a mechanic and transform mechanics into art (as any expert mechanic of material things does, consciously or unconsciously). Or one can begin as an artist and also learn the mechanics or techniques which enable fuller expression in the art. Both are essential to the total development of Jin Shin Do. And both are fun!

Becoming Aware of the Hara

In our bodies, the great center of harmony between the yang and the yin ki is the "hara," or "tanden."[1] Located approximately two fingers' width below the navel internally, the hara is our center of vital energy. Development of the hara is one of the primary secrets of Taoist inner alchemy, for it is a key to the "radiant health" of the ancient sages. As the hara is cultivated, a storehouse of ki is developed. Through this storehouse—or treasure-house—all the energy flows of the body are filled with new ki, with vital life energy. Cultivating the hara means learning to absorb, accumulate, and concentrate the ki.

According to the Taoist masters, this centering and vitalizing process must precede learning to direct the ki, either to different parts of one's own body or to others. Therefore, becoming aware of and beginning to develop the hara is the first part of the channeling process. One of the easiest ways to become aware of the hara and begin to fill this center with ki is a simple Taoist yogic meditation called "hara breathing."

There are stories of Taoist masters who, after years of practicing this and more advanced meditations, were able to do things we would regard as "magical." One traditional test of Kung Fu students in northern China, and of Zen monks in Japan, was actually melting a block of ice by sitting on it. (An alternative was swimming in the ocean in winter—but only after adequate preparation!) This was said to be possible through kindling the "Golden Stove" (or warming activities) of the hara. If you live in a climate which has cold winters, or even just cold evenings, you can experiment with "hara

[1]"Tanden" and "hara" are Japnese; "Dan Jun" is Korean; "Tan T'ien" is Chinese.

breathing" in a very practical way. A real sensation of inner warmth can be felt after just a couple minutes of this concentration, once you have practiced it enough. You will probably not wish to shed your warm overcoat, but you may find that the cold winds do not seem to penetrate through it so easily, and that the cold is actually enjoyable.

Masters of any traditional oriental health art were able to center themselves physically and emotionally much more quickly than the average man, even under extreme conditions such as attack. Aikido masters, for instance, could divert would-be attackers with just the power of their ki, using no resistance and little if any force. Ancient echoes of space age heroes! This degree of control requires years of disciplined effort. But hara breathing meditation is such a strong technique that even a short amount of practice produces many beneficial effects, and enables one to relax and center more easily in difficult and stressful situations. It also re-energizes both body and mind, and is a great pick-me-up as well as an aid to greater physical and mental freedom! Hara breathing is a very practical tool with which we can improve the quality of our daily lives.

Positions for Hara Breathing Meditation

The "hara breathing" meditation can be performed standing, sitting, or lying down—or as a series of these three postures. Any number of hand positions may be used. A few are given below, but if you wish you may use another position with which you are familiar. In any position, it is important that your shoulders and arms—and indeed your entire body—remain relaxed. Therefore, you may wish to start with a posture that most facilitates your relaxation—that is, with one that feels good!

Figure 1, in which the entire palmar surfaces of both hands are touching, and Figure 2, in which the palms rest on the sides of the rib-cage, are easiest to use in a standing or sitting position. Figure 3, with the right hand on top of the left hand and the left palm resting over the hara region, may be used standing, sitting, or lying down.

In sitting, you may use the cross-legged or half-lotus positions. Or you may kneel in the traditional Japanese "sitting" position, legs folded under the body and knees slightly

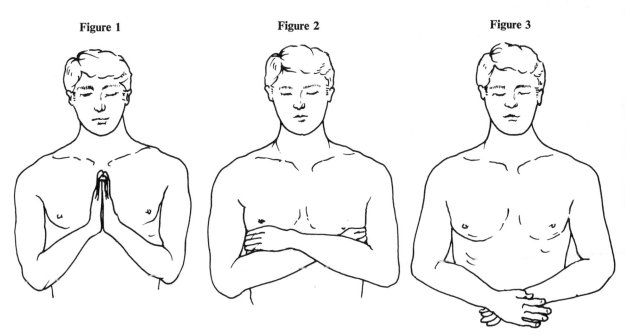

Figure 1   Figure 2   Figure 3

44

apart. The feet may be crossed so that the toes of one foot rest on top of the toes of the other. (See illustrations in Figures 4, 5, and 6.) To make these sitting or kneeling positions more comfortable, a small cushion such as the traditional Japanese *zafu* may be used. If all of these positions are still uncomfortable, you may just sit on a chair at first. However, if you maintain any position for even a few minutes at first, it will gradually become comfortable as your muscles loosen up.

In any sitting position, try to maintain an erect posture throughout the meditation time. You may wish to concentrate your attention on the hara, the center about two fingers' width below the navel, and then imagine your body arising from this center. The hara should be your center of gravity. If the inclination to slouch becomes irresistible, after a few minutes go into the lying down position. This is not just a last recourse, but also a very powerful position for developing and nourishing the hara. In fact, probably the easiest way to begin hara breathing is to lie down, using the hand position shown in Figure 3.

A pleasant and effective meditation pattern is to begin by standing and using the hand position of Figure 1, then after several minutes sit using the hand position of Figure 2, and finally lie down using the hand position of Figure 3. After a while, you may go to sleep in the last position. This just means that your body needs the revitalization of ki that occurs during sleep. The sleep that follows meditation will be very deep and refreshing.

> "*Attain to the goal of absolute vacuity;*
> *Keep to the state of perfect peace . . .*
> *Going back to the origin is called peace . . .*"[1]

Eventually, you can learn to use the "hara breathing" technique at any time and place,

as a means of helping to calm the emotions, still the mind, and both relax and re-vitalize the body. However, it is easier at first to find the peace and stillness of the inner Spirit when surrounded by outer peace and stillness or tranquil sounds. Therefore, begin by choosing a quiet place, especially one where you feel relaxed and where you won't be interrupted. Wear loose clothing and avoid eating just before practicing hara breathing meditation (but don't be overly hungry either), so that you will be physically comfortable.

Now, in your chosen position, close your eyes and begin to breathe slowly in and out through the chest. While you inhale, feel the spaces between your ribs expanding as the lungs are filled with air. As you exhale, completely let go so as to breathe out completely. After a couple of minutes, begin to breathe more deeply and slowly, focussing your attention on the hara. The phrases "Golden Stove," "Field of Elixir (of Immortality)," and "Center of Vital Energy" are descriptions of the hara which may help you to experience its nature. But the primary thing is just to concentrate on and keep your attention within the hara.

Concentrating Ki in the Center of Vitality

Control of the breath is fundamentally important in Taoist yoga meditation. "Can you regulate the breath and become soft and pliant like an infant?"[2] Continue to keep your eyes closed and to focus on the hara, the center of vitality. Keep your eyes closed during the entire meditation, in order to avoid diverting your ki outwardly or being distracted by outer things. The basic hara

---

[1] *Tao Teh Ching*, from Chapter XVI.
[2] *Ibid.*, from Chapter X.

breathing pattern is:

1. INHALE →	2. HOLD →	3. EXHALE
through the nose, expanding the hara (slow count to 5)	accumulate ki in the hara (slow count to 5)	through the mouth, contracting the hara (slow count to 5)

Read the following descriptions of each step before you begin practicing, unless you are already familiar with this technique. Don't memorize; just understand the basic principles involved. If you like, tape some of the directions and images so that you can listen to them as you practice the first few times.

1) The breathing should be gentle, so that if you held a feather or a piece of rice paper in front of your nose and mouth, it would hardly move. Having the top of the tongue resting on the roof of the mouth (in order to connect the front and back parts of the central energy channel), inhale slowly and gently through the nose. As you inhale, slowly count 1–2–3–4–5. During the entire inhalation, use your imagination or creative will to visualize the ki in the breath descending to and filling the hara.

This creative visualization, or "yi," is considered to be a necessary element of Taoist meditation. Yi is a very real force; to an incredible degree that which we actively visualize comes to exist (especially if it coincides with that which we need). Therefore, whether or not you believe that by hara breathing meditation you can kindle a "Golden Stove" within your body, just visualize the activities of the ki as directed, use your yi to concentrate your ki in the hara, and see what happens!

As you practice expanding the lower abdomen on the inhalation, the hara will naturally fill with ki. Have no fear that your lower abdomen, or "belly," will actually become expanded, however. What will happen is that the muscles of your abdomen will be tonified and will become stronger through the practice of hara breathing. You will be teaching them to relax (during the inhalation) and also to contract, but not become tense (during the exhalation).

Part of what is happening physically as you inhale "into your hara" is that your lungs are expanding downward. Your diaphragm—the muscular partition between chest and abdomen that is the most important mechanical factor in respiration—moves downward, thus enlarging the chest and drawing air into the lungs, as well as displacing the abdominal organs so that the abdomen ("belly") expands outward.

If your abdomen is remaining rigid, or not moving very much as you practice this technique, inhale again and this time use your "yi" or creative visualization to relax the diaphragm so that it can move downward more easily. As you inhale, visualize the area around your lower ribs relaxing. Pretend that it is all light, all loose, all transparent. As you visualize a downward movement from this area, you will feel your abdomen expanding of itself.

Thinking down is important. In our usual breathing we tend to fill the lungs with air in an upward motion, concentrating energy in the neck and shoulder region and increasing the tension and ki blockage that so many of us have developed in this area. Hara breathing, on the other hand, allows the parasympathetic nervous system to control our state of being, so that the responses of relaxation are encouraged. By visualizing a downward movement of vital energy into the hara on the inhalation, the ki will accumulate in its natural storehouse—the hara. It may be helpful to simply imagine that you are filling a pitcher with water—the water goes to the bottom first!

46

2) After inhaling in this way, hold the ki within the hara for the same slow count to five. This allows the ki you have concentrated in the hara to accumulate, warming and kindling the "Golden Stove." You should feel no physical tension during this "holding;" it is not like holding or repressing your breath and should not require physical effort. Just focus your attention on the hara, or continue to keep your attention there, and imagine the ki accumulating in and developing this center.

The holding step just allows the ki to revitalize the hara region and, from there, the entire body. Drawing the ki into the hara is very helpful just by itself, but once we have done this we may as well let it have a chance to work there. If at first this holding or accumulating step is difficult, if you feel a lot of tension that you cannot visualize away, then shorten the holding time as much as is necessary. Hold just a little longer than is comfortable, counting to two or three rather than to five. Or just skip this step at first; I often have clients begin hara breathing with just the inhalation and exhalation steps. As you become comfortable with these steps, add the holding step and then gradually increase the holding time until it is the same as the inhalation and exhalation.

In even this basic Taoist meditative process, we are inevitably releasing physical and emotional armoring which has prevented our complete absorption and use of both breath and ki. In hara breathing we are releasing tension in our internal organs, which can be just as constricted and armored (tense) as our external musculature. If this armor has been a long time forming, the body and mind may resist its disintegration out of habit. Therefore, it is best and actually fastest in the long run to be somewhat gentle with yourself, while being persistent in the process of gradually unfolding your inner nature and

powers.

3) During the third stage of the breathing, the exhalation, the attention should still remain focussed on the hara. Feel as though your consciousness is moving out of your head (where most of us spend entirely too much time, either in rationalizing or in worrying) and into your hara. Remove your tongue from your palate and exhale slowly through the mouth, with the lips just slightly parted. Again, remember that the exhalation should be quiet and gentle. You should not feel the air moving in front of your face. As you count to five, contract your lower abdomen so as to exhale completely.

With your hands on the lower abdomen in the position shown in Figure 3 on page 43, you should feel your hands moving up and down as your abdomen expands on the inhalation and contracts on the exhalation. Having your hands in this position will enable you to concentrate more easily on the hara and to be more aware of this movement; therefore, you may assume this position whenever you are having difficulty freeing your breathing. After the exhalation, immediately begin the cycle again, keeping a smooth and continuous rhythm. There is no holding time after the exhalation. Continue the inhale-hold-exhale pattern throughout the meditation time. Of course, you may stop counting when the rhythm is established.

Mental Attitudes and Meditation

When you actually begin to meditate, do not allow the details of these steps to concern you too much. The most important thing during the entire basic pattern of inhaling to five, holding to five (or less at first), and exhaling to five, is to concentrate your attention on the hara itself and not on techniques, except as a means to this end. As you meditate you may feel a sense of warmth in the hara, or a sense of freeness and energy fullness. However, again, do not stay your attention on what you might experience or on whether your experience is adequate; simply concentrate on and visualize your hara. As long as you seek growth, your experiencing is always adequate.

As thoughts or pictures come into your mind, treat them neither like enemies nor like friends. If you actively try to expel them, they will be the focus of your attention as surely as if you wished them to be. Allow them to enter and exit your consciousness freely, for if you resist their entry they will come anyway—and stay longer. In meditation, you will meet and melt away emotional and mental blocks, as well as physical tensions and armoring, by reaching out to contact Nature and by reaching in to contact and center in your Inner Nature.

There is an old Taoist story which clarifies this process to me. A master and his disciple went on a long journey. They were monks, and monks were not supposed to touch females in any way or at any time. At one point, however, they met a young and beautiful girl on the banks of a muddy and turbulent stream. The master, seeing her plight, picked her up on his back and carried her over the water. That evening, after the two had gone quite a way further on their journey, the disciple finally had the courage to ask, "Master, how is it that you carried the young woman, when we are not supposed to deal with females?" The master replied, "Disciple, how is it that you are still carrying that woman? I put her down on the other side of the stream."

You will generally feel peaceful and refreshed, high and happy, after meditating. However, it is not uncommon to sometimes also feel a bit grouchy or unsettled after you

first begin meditating. This is because you are expelling stagnant ki that has been locked into your physical structure. As it is released, you experience it on a more conscious level, whereas formerly it colored your experience on a subconscious level.

Both expelling and developing are necessary. You cannot grow without also letting go. This letting go, or expelling, may be a catharsis—a fairly intense release of the emotions and of the physical armoring. Or it may be a more continuous letting go of one little thing after another, in the process of living life five minutes at a time. Growth—not into something or someone different from what we are, but into the Free Spirits we already potentially or internally are—can take place in big spurts or else in little continuous ways. Thus the oriental masters described *satori*, or enlightenment, as a state of being which can be realized in a flash or in a series of little flashes. It is like climbing a gradual staircase: one step up and then a plateau, then again one step up. (Or maybe a couple of steps up, one step back, and then a plateau!) If you look only for the big flashes, you may miss the little ones.

"Hara breathing" is the fundamental Taoist yogic meditation and ki-development technique. There are many variant ki-development and ki-directing techniques which can be practiced after this basic breathing pattern begins to feel natural. Though many of these techniques are essentially simple, they are also very strong and the details of their practice are important. Therefore, they should not be learned just from books. However, as long as the above instructions are understood and followed, the student will be able to gain much from just the basic hara breathing technique.

It is highly beneficial to meditate in this way for from fifteen to thirty minutes (or longer) once or twice a week—or as often as you wish. You may sometimes want to do hara breathing for a few minutes before doing a Jin Shin Do treatment, or else after doing one or more treatments. Doing hara breathing in the lying down position is also a good way to relax yourself into a deeper and more refreshing sleep at night.

Using the Hands to Channel Ki

In the "hara breathing" meditation, you have tapped the great ocean of ki, absorbing this universal spiritual energy more fully and concentrating it within yourself. Concentrating the ki in the hara is the first part of channeling ki to others. The second part, the actual process of directing this ki through the hands, is very simple and only requires using your yi, your creative visualization.

After you have done the hara breathing for a few minutes, you can try the basic channeling pattern. Sit on a chair, placing your palms on your thighs. Breathe slowly and gently, with the pattern of inhaling to the count of five and exhaling to the count of five. You need not hold the ki in the hara during channeling.

As you inhale, feel the ki in the breath concentrating in the hara as you did in "hara breathing." As you exhale, visualize the energy accumulated in the hara flowing up the midline of the torso to the region of the heart center, or chakra. Here, in the residence of Shin, your compassion or desire to help someone else will focus the ki. Then visualize the ki flowing down the arms and channel the ki through the palms. (This route is illustrated in the diagram below.) Repeat this inhalation-exhalation pattern several times.

Thus the basic channeling pattern is:

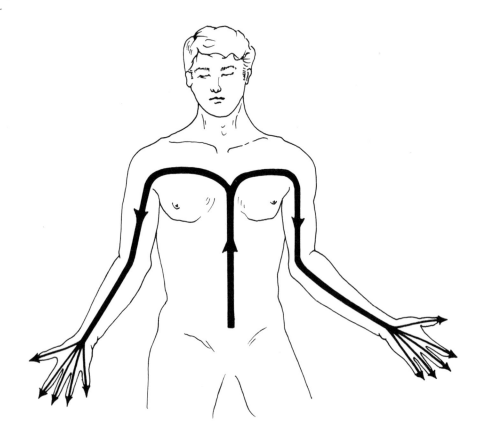

1. INHALE $\longrightarrow$ 2. EXHALE

| (through the nose, concentrating ki in the hara) | (through the nose, channeling ki through the hands) |

After you have done this for a couple of minutes, you will feel your palms becoming warmer. The muscles of your thighs will relax as they receive this strong new ki from your hands. If a friend or pet is available, you can now try channeling this energy into another being. Place your palms on the hara region, back, chest, forehead, or any other area. As you inhale, concentrate the ki in your hara; as you exhale, channel it out through your palms into the area you are touching. (After you begin doing treatments, channel the ki through your palms or, usually, fingertips.) You may visualize that area being released from physical or emotional tensions, and being filled with fresh, vibrant new ki.

While giving a Jin Shin Do treatment, use this channeling pattern as a re-charging process, rather than doing it continuously. Once the tapping, accumulating, and channeling of the ki have been established by this simple breathing pattern, the treatment process itself will assure their continuance, for Jin Shin Do is an inherently meditative technique. The channeling technique mainly establishes the direction of ki flow from outside yourself, through yourself, to the other person. It allows you to more quickly and easily become a channel for the universal spiritual energy—ki.

A good way to use the channeling pattern within a treatment is to do it for a few minutes near the beginning of each treatment, and also several times within the treatment. During the treatment itself, you will of course not need to assume any special position in order to use the channeling technique. Simply practice channeling in whatever position you use to give the treatment, and you will begin to discover the magic in your fingertips—and the magic within you.

> "*He who knows the masculine and yet keeps to the feminine*
> *Will become a channel drawing all the world towards it;*
> *Being a channel of the world, he will not be severed from the eternal virtue,*
> *And then he can return again to the state of infancy.*"[1]

---

[1]*Tao Teh Ching*, from Chapter XXXIII.

5. THE STRANGE FLOWS OF ACUPRESSURE

The ancient oriental sages saw no real distinction between man and earth, earth and universe, microcosm and macrocosm. The same laws that operate in the macrocosm—our world and universe—also work in the microcosm—our bodies and minds. Because macrocosm and microcosm are one, looking at the former gives insight into the latter—and vice versa. "Without going out of the door, one can know the whole world; Without peeping out of the window, one can see the Tao of heaven."[1]

The people of the ancient Orient lived close to the earth and were watchful of the skies. They saw in the dynamic changes of nature reflections of the Tao: that profound truth which includes nature's flux yet is beyond that flux, as the whole is greater than its parts. They saw themselves clearly as offspring of the Tao, subject to the same laws and principles that all of nature followed without deviation.

Due to the antiquity of their civilization, the Chinese were among the first to develop a logical theory of organic functioning, looking at life from the perspective of life forces and energy flow. Their theories have withstood the test of time and are still the basis of modern acupuncture and acupressure. If we put ourselves into their situation 5000 years ago, understanding the basic philosophies of their civilization that we have already discussed, we can see how the oriental system of therapeutics and health arts might have arisen.

Imagine that you are a peasant of ancient China, living where your ancestors have lived for centuries. It has been a very dry growing season. The lake at the center of the valley, upon which the village has relied throughout the season for water, has fallen to the lowest watermark that your grandfather can remember. The rice paddies are drying out, so that a poor harvest is dreaded. All the village have been beseeching Kuan Yin, goddess of compassion, to send rain for the fields, for the animals, for the people —for life.[2]

Finally, the rains come. For several days the life-gift of the heavens pours to the earth. The earth absorbs what it can, streams fill, ponds form, and excess water drains from these into the lake—the valley's natural reservoir. The lake rises higher and higher. Will drought now turn to flooding, equally an evil for the land? But no: this wonderful reservoir sends its abundance through adjoining channels and rivers, reaching at last another lake in another valley. Even though the rains did not reach its drought-stricken people, the excess rainfall of your region has followed the earth's natural waterways to both relieve your village of its surplus, and at

---

[1] *Tao Teh Ching*, from Chapter XLVIII.
[2] Kuan Yin is not necessary taken to represent an actual goddess, but may instead be seen as a symbol of compassion energy.

the same time send that surplus where there was a need.

The philosophers and doctors of the villages rejoice along with the farmers and craftsmen and merchants. Reflecting on this natural phenomenon they wonder: might there not be a similar system of reservoirs, of flow and of flood control, within the human body as well? Excess energy can build up in parts of the body just as excess water can rise in the lakes and rivers of the earth. How does the body take care of its excess? Periods of energy deficiency occur in the body. Could there be reservoirs that store surplus body energy to meet such situations?

From meditation and from the experience of treating the human body in all its states of distress, what they discovered was an analogous and wondrous system of lakes, channels, rivers and streams within the human body. Through these pathways the vital energy (ki) of the body flows to every part of the body, nourishing and harmonizing the whole.

Rivers and Streams in the Body

The body's rivers are the twelve "organ meridians"—so-called because each is connected with and gives energy to a particular organ and set of correlative functions. Through these meridians, the vital energies of heaven and earth communicate with and flow through us, nourishing every nerve and every blood vessel, every muscle and every bone, every organ and every gland, every tissue and every system of the entire body.

We absorb the heaven and earth ki directly, through various vital centers in the body. We also absorb the yang ki of heaven through the breath and the yin ki of earth through our food. These energies combine in the human body and are transformed into the bodily ki,

which flows through the twelve great rivers or meridians and their tributaries. Together, these rivers and streams form a continuous route which covers the entire body, flowing both externally and internally.

Oriental therapeutic philosophy says that if the ki flow through the twelve meridians is smooth and unimpeded, and if each meridian receives a balanced amount of ki, then the functioning of the body is harmonious.[1] But if the ki flow stagnates, or is blocked or impeded, then harmony turns to disharmony, and disharmony to dis-ease.

What can cause this ki stagnation? Traumatic experiences, difficult environments, improper use or dis-use of body mobility, low-quality food, polluted air, extreme climatic conditions, and a whole host of other tension-forming things—combined with lack of body-mind awareness. As alone as we might feel in our problems, no one has a monopoly on physical or emotional tension (or the accompanying ki stagnation). Even spiritual masters sometimes have a few tense or blocked points. Have you ever met anybody who was "perfect" and totally hassle-free?

But there are people who are generally happy and basically enjoy life, feeling free more often than not. How do they do it? Usually, they are more aware of their own physical, emotional, and spiritual condition. They enjoy experiencing being and desire to grow, so they are receptive to new ways of thinking and acting, to new feelings and thoughts. Having faith in themselves, in their own ability to grow and change, they can make the most of any situation that arises. Even tension and ki stagnation can be

---

[1]It is not the purpose of this book to describe each of the twelve organ meridians. Instead, we will be learning about another set of energy flows (the body's "channels") which regulate and balance all of the organ meridians, in addition to nourishing the vital centers.

appreciated, for in learning to release these we can learn more about ourselves and about life.

Whenever we try to stop the cycle of growth, not letting go of the past and so not fully experiencing and enjoying the moment, each problem and tension that we hold onto multiplies in effect. Like a series of reflecting mirrors, the body reflects the ki flow, the emotions reflect the body, the mind reflects the emotions, and the spirit reflects the mind. Looking the other way, the mind reflects the spirit, the emotions reflect the mind, the body reflects the emotions, and the ki flow reflects the body. All these aspects are one; therefore, any influence is multi-dimensional.

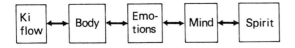

The ancient acupressure technique used in Jin Shin Do is a wonderful helper for the times when, due to pressure and difficulties, we find it difficult to let go spontaneously. Instead of allowing ki blockage and tension to get out of hand and destroy our feeling of physical and emotional well-being (or to help recover that feeling!), we can facilitate and speed our own recovery and that of others.

Lakes and Channels in the Body

Just as the earth has a system for storing water to use in deficient periods and for sending excess water from one area into another, so the body also has a system for dealing with deficiencies and excesses of ki. This system of eight channels is the basis of much Taoist yoga practice and of ancient systems of acupressure and acupuncture which, though little known in the West, are respected by oriental masters. To some

people, of course, all of the energy flow routes or meridians will seem strange at first. However, even to the ancient Chinese this set of eight extra meridians were wondrous and amazing, and thus they were called the "Strange Flows."

Through these eight "Strange Flows" all of the energy flows of the body are inter-related.[1] This truly marvelous system regulates the energy in and adjusts the functions of all the body's rivers and streams and, through them, the entire body. Like a series of lakes and channels, the Strange Flows act as reservoirs of energy for the body and its meridians, balancing out excesses and deficiencies of energy throughout the system. We will discuss each of the four pairs of Strange Flows individually: the Great Central Channel (Vessel of Conception or Jen Mo, and Governing Vessel or Tu Mo): the Great Regulator Channel (Yin and Yang Wei Mo); the Great Bridge Channel (Yin and Yang Chiao Mo); and the Penetrating and Belt Channels (Ch'ang Mo and Tai Mo).

Why are these flows so strange? First of all, with the exceptions of the Vessel of Conception and Governing Vessel (the Great Central Channel), the Strange Flows do not have particular points of their own belonging only to themselves, as do all the twelve organ meridians. Instead, they are somewhat like the catbird, which creates no nests of its own but uses those of other birds. All of their points are points which belong to and are on the twelve organ meridians (and, to a limited degree, the Conception and Governing Vessels, where these intersect the other Strange Flows). Their points are points at which the organ meridians cross the flow

[1]Sometimes translated: "Wondrous Flows," "Extraordinary Channels," "Odd Conduits," or "Psychic Channels"—all of which give clues to their nature. Also sometimes called, simply, "extra meridians."

routes of the Strange Flows.

Secondly, again with the exceptions of the Conception and Governing Vessels, the ki does not flow continuously through the Strange Flows as it does through the twelve organ meridians. Instead, the ki flows through these extra vessels when there is a need for the body to adjust the balance of energy flow in the rivers and streams (the meridians and their tributaries). Because of this difference, the Strange Flows are referred to as "channels" or "conduits" to distinguish them from the organ "meridians."

How do the eight Strange Flows regulate the energy in the twelve organ meridians? Following the diagram below, suppose that there is an excess of ki in one of the arm meridians ①. Suppose that tension and excess ki builds up at a point along its route ②. When this excess begins to overflow, it goes into the adjoining Strange Flow ③. Following this pathway, the excess eventually arrives at an area and point ④ which is deficient. From there, if the need exists, the excess can flow into the related organ meridian ⑤.

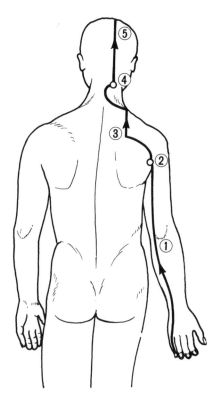

If this regulating system of eight strange or psychic channels were always functioning properly, there would be no problem. They would continuously adjust and regulate the twelve organ meridians. These would be balanced, their ki flow would be smooth and unimpeded, and the body would be harmonious.

However, just as beavers may build a dam on an earthly river or channel, so the beavers of personal and cultural tension may build dams—tension or armoring—on the channels of the body. If these dams are small, and if the energy flow through the channels is reasonably strong, then these dams will be washed away by the normal flow of the ki before they become large obstacles. But if we do not let go of physical and emotional tensions soon enough, more and more tension builds at various points. The dams grow too big, and the flow of energy too weak, for the balancing channels (the "Strange Flows") to function efficiently. At this time, the body needs a little help. This is the function of Jin Shin Do.

The Strange Flows are strongly and easily affected by the hands and by meditation—hence their alternate name, "Psychic Channels." Because of this, and because of their vital regulatory functions, the Strange Flows are the foundation of the Jin Shin Do point and treatment system. (Of course, the organ meridians and in fact all the principles of acupuncture are also used; they are considered even in the basic treatment patterns and are increasingly used by the student as he or she advances.) Through the release and re-balancing of Jin Shin Do treatments, and through the growing awareness of body and mind that develops when giving and receiving these treatments, we can help the body to help itself.

Direction of Ki Flow through the Eight Channels

The ki can flow through these channels in any direction as it leaves a point of excess and flows through the reservoir to a point or area of deficiency. However, for the Strange Flows to balance the entire body during a Jin Shin Do treatment, the ki flow through the Strange Flow channels must be continuous and smooth. Therefore, in the formerly secret Taoist yogic techniques and esoteric acupressure forms, the Great Central Channel and the other Strange Flows were directed up the back and down the front.

In acupuncture texts, on the other hand, the Great Central Channel (the most well-known of the Strange Flows) and the others are shown going up the back and up the front. Reasons for this difference could be explained in much esoteric detail, but basically the feeling is that the latter is in fact the usual or average (adequate) condition, whereas the former is a condition which should be normal and can be evolved.

Noting that flowing up the back and front directs the ki towards the head—the brain and sense organs—it is easy to understand why the Taoist masters called this an emphasis on "latter life." They teach that before birth, we receive nourishment through the "Gate of Former Life"—the umbilicus, of which the hara is a vestige. After birth, we receive nourishment through the "Gate of Latter Life"—the mouth. Gradually, the influence of the hara decreases as intelligence develops and cultural habit patterns are established. These also begin to sway the heart center, residence of Shin. The light of the spiritual consciousness, residing in the "third eye," dims.

Directing the flows up the back and down the front was viewed as a return to "former life"—the freedom aspired to by seekers—and therefore as the most powerful way of replenishing the entire body energy. It also encourages a more continuous release of blocks and allows the released ki to more easily flow wherever it is needed.

The eight Strange Flows are traditionally grouped into four pairs. Each pair consists of two flows, or channels, with complimentary functions and routes. The functions of each pair are given in the remainder of this chapter. The numbers next to points on the charts refer to the thirty main Jin Shin Do points that we will be learning. Do not be concerned about finding them while first reading this section, as each point will be described in detail in the next chapter.

Great Regulator Channel (Yin and Yang Wei Mo)

According to the classics, the Regulator acts as "the binding network of all the vessels." The yin part, going along the front of the body, connects with all of the yin organ meridians—the spleen, liver, kidney, lung, pericardium, and heart meridians. The yang part, going along the back and through the head, connects with all of the yang organ meridians—the stomach, gall bladder, bladder, large intestine, triple warmer (which governs energy production), and small intestine meridians.

Like a linking net, the Regulator thus connects with all twelve organ meridians. It acts to maintain and adjust their basic functions through its control of the nourishing and defensive energies of the body. The yin Regulator "moves all the yin," controls the nourishing energy of the body, and regulates the blood, as well as the interior regions of the body. The yang Regulator "moves all the yang," controls the defense energy of the body, and regulates the resistance (to external "evils") as well as the exterior regions of the body. Thus the classics say that "when the Yang Wei Mo (yang Regulator) is imbalanced, the person suffers from colds and fevers," while "when the yin wei mo (yin Regulator) is diseased, the person suffers from heart pains."[1]

In many respects, all of the Strange Flows are like parents, while the organ meridians are like children. The Great Regulator is like the necessary disciplining or restraining aspect of parenthood, subtly and smoothly regulating the children's activities so as to support and sustain each one individually, and also guiding the children's interactions so as to maintain harmonious communication and cooperation between them all.

---

[1]Obviously, there could be many other causes of heart pains.

The Great Regulator Channel: Yin Wei Mo（陰維脈）and Yang Wei Mo（陽維脈）

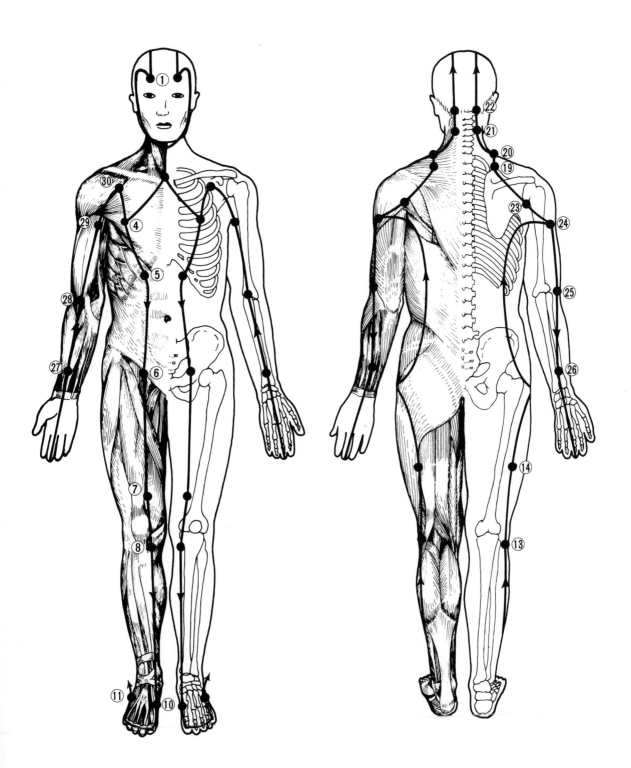

The Great Bridge Channel: Yin Chiao Mo（陰蹻脈）and Yang Chiao Mo
（陽蹻脈）

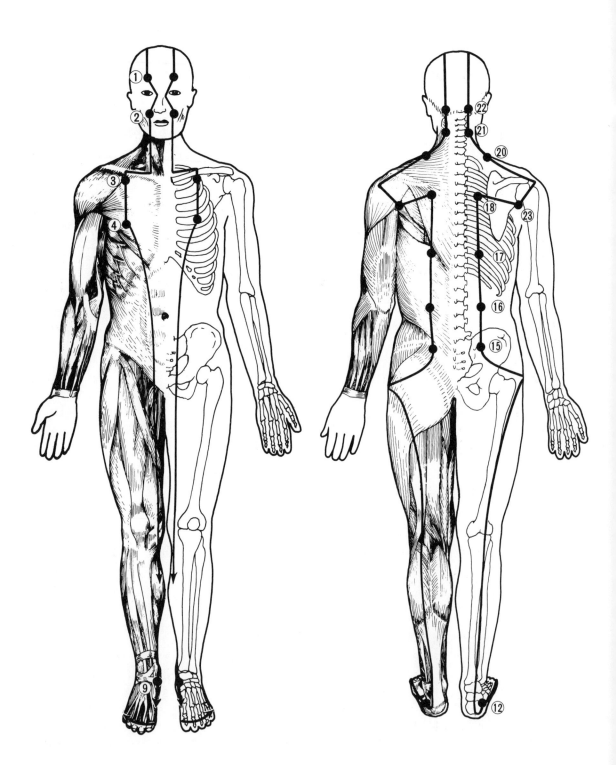

Great Bridge Channel (Yin and Yang Chiao Mo)

The Bridge Channel is like a connecting bridge linking the yin and the yang so that the proper energy balance can be maintained. It also acts as a bridge between the stored energy of the body and areas or flows which are in need of ki. The part going along the front is yin; the part going along the back is yang.

The classics say, "When the yin chi is deficient, yang chi is abundant and there is often insomnia. When the yang chi is deficient, yin chi is abundant and one is often very sleepy." This means that an excess in one part of this channel is usually accompanied by deficient energy in the other. Yang ki (or chi) is active, assertive energy, so when it is in excess (when the yang Bridge Channel is blocked) there may be excess activity and the inability to sleep. Yin ki is passive, receptive energy, so when it is in excess (when the yin Bridge Channel is blocked) there may be fatigue and drowsiness. Excess of ki is usually accompanied by tension, which is a blockage of ki.

Because of its energy-balancing functions, this pair of flows was traditionally used for persons with hyper- or hypo-tension. Because it is also related to the heels, another traditional use was to increase the speed of runners.

The Bridge Channel is like the nourishing aspect of parenthood, for it most strongly regulates the amounts of energy remaining in and being used by each meridian. Like a wise parent, it attempts to assure that this nourishment is properly balanced, so that each child receives the proportion of yin and yang energy which best suits its development.

Great Central Channel (Jen Mo and Tu Mo)

The Central Channel is the most primal of all the energy flows. The two parts of the channel are the Vessel of Conception (from below the mouth down the median line of the front) and the Governing Vessel (from the coccyx up the spinal column and along the median line over the head down to below the nose). The Conception Vessel is the "sea" of all the yin meridians. Sometimes called the "Great Mother Flow," it is the strongest yin of all the energy flows. The Governing Vessel is the "sea" of all the yang meridians. Sometimes called the "Great Father Flow," it is the strongest yang of all the energy flows. The Great Central Channel as a whole is so vital to the body's well-being that it is considered to be the ruling energy channel of the body and spirit.

All of the organ meridians receive energy from and give excess energy into this pair of flows. All of the yang meridians are connected to the Central Channel at some point(s) along the Governing Vessel, and all of the yin meridians are connected to it at some point(s) along the Conception Vessel. It is through these central meeting points

The Great Central Channel: Jen Mo（任脉）and Tu Mo（督脉）

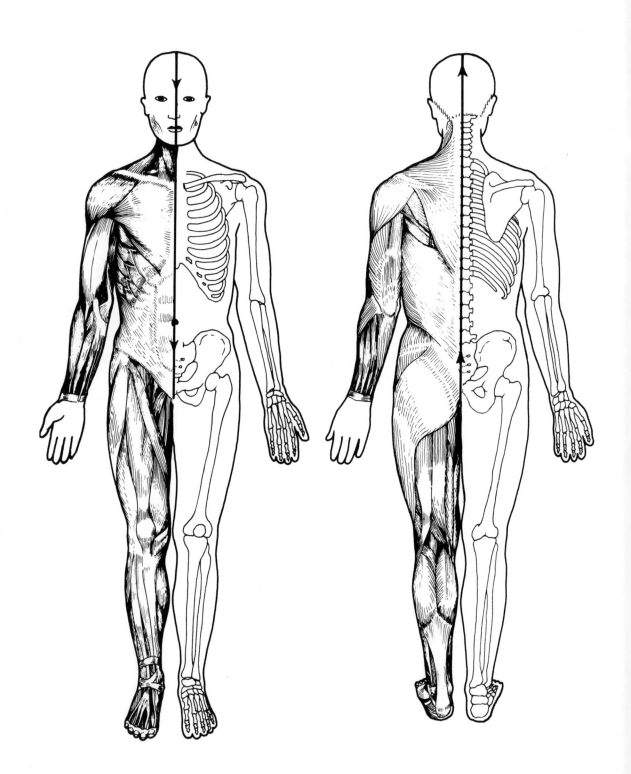

that the left and right sides of each bilateral meridian are connected to each other and are able to form one continuous flow.

The Conception Vessel influences the lower abdomen and, as its name implies, the reproductive functions. The Governing Vessel influences the spine, and helps determine the constitution by regulating the native or pre-natal energy. Perhaps most importantly, this pair of Strange Flows has especially strong psychic functions. The Conception Vessel influences the state of spiritual peace or unrest, while the Governing Vessel influences the state of nervous stability or instability.

The Vessel of Conception and Governing Vessel do have points of their own (for diagram see page 117) as well as a continuous energy flow—characteristics of the twelve organ meridians not exhibited by the other Strange Flows. Though they are listed with the twelve organ meridians in many modern books, traditionally this pair belongs to the Strange Flows because of its very strong activities of equalizing and regulating the overall body ki.

Penetrating and Belt Channels: (Ch'ang Mo and Tai Mo)

These two channels are in some ways the oddest of the Strange Flow couples. The other three pairs are like front and back, not only physically but also in terms of their yin-yang balancing functions. These two, on the other hand, have rather individual functions and flow routes.

The Penetrating Channel, called the "sea of the twelve meridians," stores the true body ki. It helps to regulate the development

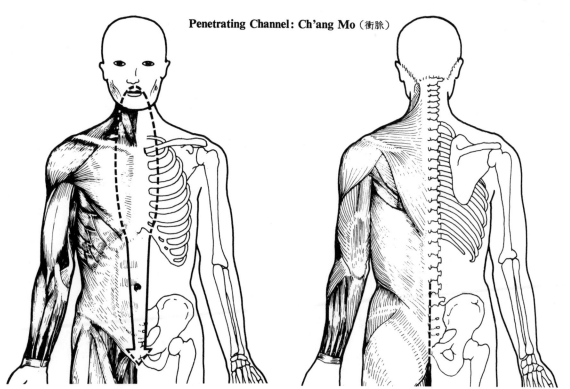

Penetrating Channel: Ch'ang Mo （衝脈）

62

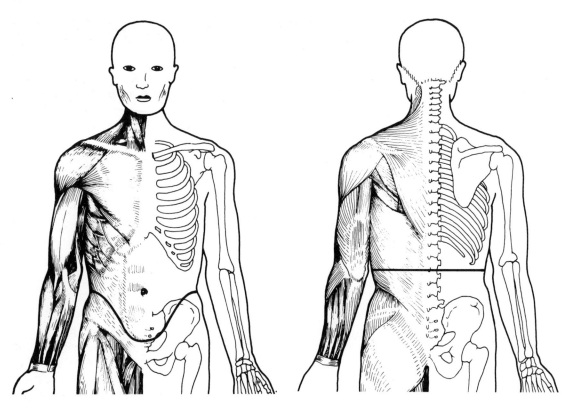

Belt Channel: Tai Mo（帯脈）

of both pre-natal and post-natal energy or ki. The classics say the Penetrating Channel "restrains and regulates the sinews and meridians of the whole body." Also called the "sea of blood," it has regulating connections with the uterus and with the meridians governing the female functions.

According to Taoist yoga, the Governing Vessel, Conception Vessel, and Penetrating Channel are the three great psychic channels, connecting the vital centers from the root to the crown. "From them radiates an intricate network of minor channels by means of which cosmic energy (prana)[1] can be transmitted throughout the body, being achieved principally by yogic breathing."[2] Releasing

and directing ki through these channels generally has a calming and spiritually uplifting effect.

The Belt Channel is the only energy flow in the body which during its entire course flows horizontally, rather than vertically or diagonally. It is like a belt slung around the hips, regulating and equalizing all of the meridians which flow through the back, front, and sides of the torso. The Belt Channel has special regulating functions for the abdominal region, our physical center.

[1]Indian term for ki.
[2]*The Secret and the Sublime: Taoist Mysteries and Magic*, by John Blofeld, Dutton, New York, 1973, page 141.

6. DISCOVERING THIRTY MAIN ACU-POINTS

Jin Shin Do acupressure, while it can include many additional specific points as the student progresses, is based on the primary use of just thirty bilateral points. These are all points of the eight Strange Flows, and they are all important acupuncture points, as well as points at which tension and ki blockage commonly occur. Through working on these points, the Strange Flows and thus the energic body can be regulated. The release and smooth functioning of these points is very important to the body, mind, emotions, and spirit.

In addition to these points, we will occasionally be choosing among about fifteen of the unilateral points of the Great Central Channel. These central points will be easily found by anatomical landmarks, and so will not be included in the descriptions given in this chapter.

How do you find the thirty main points? The simplest and most fundamental method of locating acu-points is by how they feel. Anatomical landmarks are also important, and will be given for each point. Once your fingertips are in the area described, the easiest way of locating the exact points is to feel for the place of greatest tension in that area. You can also feel for a slight depression or hollow at each point—a little groove in a bone, or a slight depression between muscle fibers, or between tendons and muscles. Even if you cannot find this little hollow at first, it will usually be accurate to just hold the tightest point, since these points are so frequently sites of ki blockage and tension. They are frequently sensitive to pressure when they are blocked—unless they are so tense and hard that there is very little feeling. This is especially true of all points located in very muscular areas.

How small is an acu-point? The apex of each point, or the place at which stimulation has the strongest effect, is quite tiny. But the area affected by and affecting each point is about the size of a dime. As long as you are within this area, you will be able to release and re-direct the ki. By looking for sensory informations such as those listed above, you will also be learning to feel the muscular condition and to sense the ki state while you are giving treatments. Developing the sensitivity in your fingertips in this way is one of your first missions in becoming an acupressurist. It will be an enjoyable one!

The thirty points most used in Jin Shin Do are numbered for convenience, in the order shown on the following charts. By learning this simple numbering system, the student can easily follow formulae for a great many different acupressure treatments, rather than having to memorize each individual pattern. The points can also be easily referred to and discussed. They are numbered consecutively down the front and up the back of the body, then down outside of the arms and up the inside of the arms. If you note that there are ten points on the front of the body, twelve on

Major Strange Flow Points

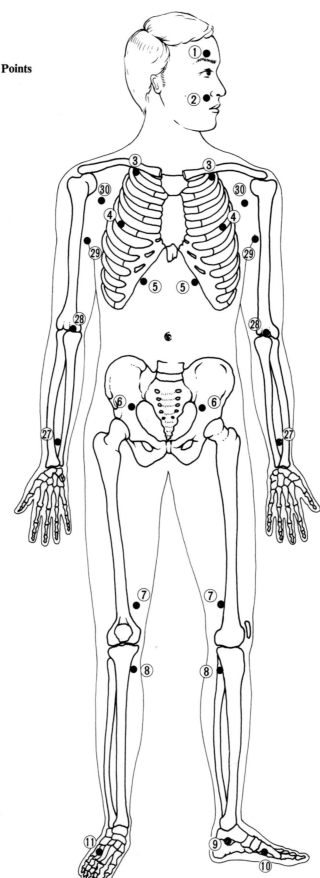

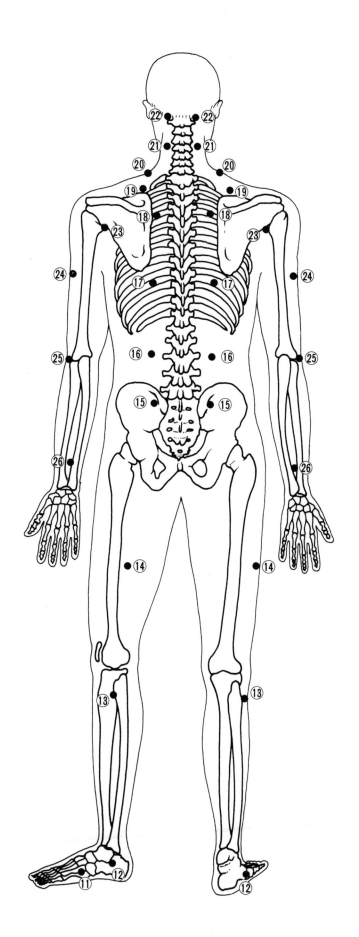

the back of the body, and eight on the arms (four on the outside of the arm and four on the inside), it will not be difficult to remember their numbering. Additionally, points will be illustrated next to each treatment pattern given in this book.

As each point is described below, its acupuncture numbering according to the accepted western numbering system will be given, in addition to its Jin Shin Do number. This is for the benefit of readers who might already be familiar with the acu-points. Readers who have not previously studied the acu-point system should simply ignore these notations, which will be given in parentheses. Decoding or memorizing them is not important to the basic practice of Jin Shin Do.

As you read the following descriptions, remember that each of these thirty main points is bilateral; it will be found in the same place on the right and left sides of the body. Try finding each point on yourself as you read the directions for locating it. If you are reading this book at the same time as a partner, friend or relative, you can try finding the points on each other and learn even more quickly by receiving feedback from the other person. It would of course be helpful to have an acupressurist or acupuncturist show you how to find each point, if you have that opportunity.

In the next chapter, we will discuss the treatment touch and practice doing some short, easy treatment patterns. For now, as you try locating the points on another person, just use a gradual firm pressure. Avoid any pressure strong enough to cause excessive sensitivity in the other person. As long as you apply pressure gradually, it will be all right to apply enough pressure to discover and feel the tension or sensitivity that may exist at some or many of these points.

Locations and Functions of the Thirty Main Jin Shin Do Treatment Points

❶ (GB 14)

This point is located on the forehead above the eyebrows. Draw a line directly up from the center of the pupil through the forehead. You will find a little hollow about a finger's width above the eyebrow. This point must be held quite gently. You may easily feel the ki here, manifesting as a subtle vibration. When the forehead is tense, as if the person is worried, you may feel a tiny wire of tension at this point. Wrinkle your brow as though you were very anxious about something, and see if you can find this wire. Be sure to relax the forehead completely afterwards!

The "number ones" strongly influence the consciousness. They help calm the spirit and

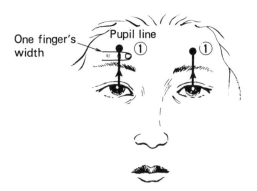

brighten the vision, and were also traditionally used to help release stiffness in the neck and facial tensions, as well as fear.

❷ (St 3)

This point is located at the bottom of the cheekbone, directly down from the center of the eye. To find it, trace a line from the nose to the outside of the cheek, along the curve of the cheekbone (line 1). Then draw another line from the center of the eye down the cheeks (line 2) until it intersects the first line. The point, which is often quite tender upon pressure, will be located at this intersection. It is held by placing the fingertips at the bottom of the cheekbone and pressing slightly upwards, onto the bone.

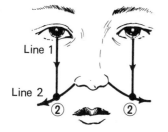

The "number twos" influence the face and clear the nasal passages. They were also traditionally used for conditions such as colds, stuffy nose, sinus problems, and toothache.[1]

❸ (St 13)

This point is located just below the collarbone (clavicle) in the space between the first and second ribs. Starting from the bony protrusion which can be felt just below the throat, trace a line along the collarbone outside to the shoulders. Divide this line approximately in half, then go below the collarbone until you feel a point that is slightly sore upon pressure.

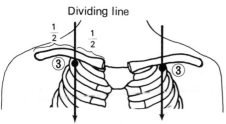

Dividing line

The "number threes" help free the breathing and encourage proper functioning of the lungs and bronchi. Their release is important for the smooth flow of many different energy flows through the chest.

❹ (St 16)

This point is located in the space between the third and fourth ribs, directly up from the nipples. Find the first rib above the breasts on a female and above the nipples on a male. Then go into the space between that rib and the next higher one. The point is often somewhat sore upon pressure, especially on females.

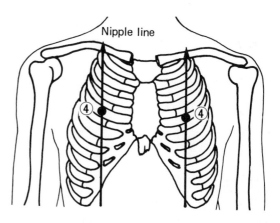

Nipple line

The "number fours" encourage proper functioning of the ki in the breast region and help promote an optimistic spirit. They were also traditionally used for heart-burn, shortness of breath, and melancholy feelings.

[1]Acupuncture is an art with a long, interesting, and important history. Therefore, historical information such as this will be given for most points, if these traditions might be interesting to the student. That a point was traditionary "used for" a given condition or area does not, however, mean that the point by itself cured the condition traditionary associated with it. In studying the acu-points, it is most important to understand their positive functions, so that they can be used to help promote "radiant health."

❺ (Lv 14)

This point is located at the junction of the ninth rib cartilage to the eighth rib. Follow the bottom of the rib-cage from the bottom of the breastbone (sternum) until you come to the first major indentation. Trace a line vertically down from the nipples, and the point should be a little inside of this line. Hold this point by placing your fingertips onto the bottom of the rib-cage and pressing slightly upward, onto the rib and not into the abdomen.

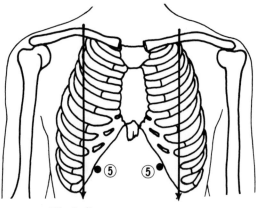

Nipple line

The "number fives" are especially important to the liver and gall bladder meridians. They also influence the diaphragm and were traditionally used for abdominal tension or uneasiness, "side aches" (as from running), belching, hiccoughs, and snoring.

❻ (Sp 13)

This point is located approximately two fingers' width above the middle of the groin. If you draw a line vertically upward from the middle of the thigh (along the crease of your slacks—or imagine one), the point will be on this line and inside of the lower edge of the pelvic bone. Some people feel ticklish or instinctively defensive at this point. If the point is held firmly, but without excessive pressure, these sensations will usually disappear quickly.

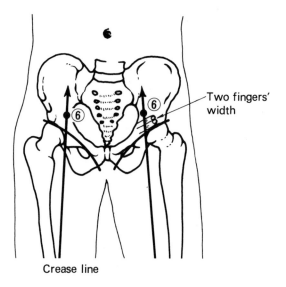

Two fingers' width

Crease line

The "number sixes" influence the tension or relaxation of the abdomen, groin, thigh, and sexual organs. They were also traditionally used for menstrual cramps, indigestion, and intestinal weakness or discomfort.

❼ (Sp 10)

This point is located about three fingers' width above the top of the knee, on the inside of the thigh. It may be easily recognized by the usual sensitivity to pressure at its site.

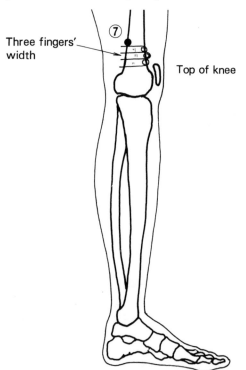

Three fingers' width

Top of knee

The "number sevens," as their name "Sea of Blood" indicates, help promote the smooth functioning of the female organs. They were traditionally used for menstrual cramps and other female problems, as well as genital problems. These points help release the thighs and knees, and were also traditionally used for indigestion and itching.

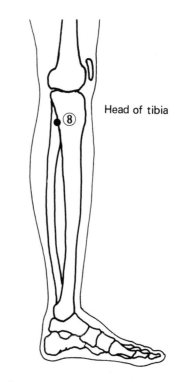

Head of tibia

⑧ (Sp 9)

This point is located on the inside of the leg just below the head, or top, of the tibia (the large bone that you will feel along the inside of the lower leg). The point may be quite tender upon pressure.

The "number eights" are very helpful for any yin body conditions. They influence the knees and legs, and were also traditionally used to help release lower back pain and bodily swelling ("water weight").

⑨ (K 6)

This point is found about a finger's width below the inner ankle bone (medial malleolus). You will find a little hollow there which may be sensitive to pressure.

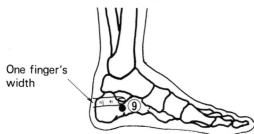

One finger's width

The "number nines" help balance the yin (anterior) Bridge Channel, and would therefore be used for drowsiness or an excessive need to sleep. As one of their names "Joyful Sleep" indicates, they encourage a deeper and more refreshing sleep. They influence the heels and the female sexual organs, as well as the kidneys. These points were also traditionally used for tiredness of the four limbs and sadness.

⑩ (Sp 4)

This point is located in a little hollow just below the metatarsal-cuneiform joint of the big toe. To find it, draw a line along the arch of your foot from the big toe "knuckle" (first metatarsal-phalanges joint) towards the heel, ending just in front of the inner ankle bone (medial malleolus). Divide this line in half and then go just below the protrusion you will feel there (the metatarsal joint). You will find a little groove which may be quite sensitive to pressure. Hold the point with your fingertips pressing up toward the metatarsal.

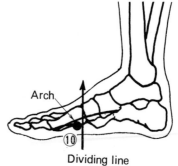

Arch

Dividing line

The "number tens" help balance the yin (anterior) Regulator and the Penetrating Channel. They influence the circulation, especially in the feet, and help to balance gaps in body energy, adjusting the flow of ki to fill deficiencies. They were traditionally used for cold feet, foot cramps, abdominal and stomach tensions, and hypochondria.

⑪ (GB 41)
This point is located on the outside of the foot, about halfway between the base of the toes and the front part of the outer ankle bone (outer malleolus). To find it, start from the space between the fourth and little toes. Follow that space (going between the fourth and fifth metatarsals) up the foot until you feel a joint. The point is located just below this joint, in the space between the fourth and fifth metatarsals. It may be somewhat sensitive to pressure.

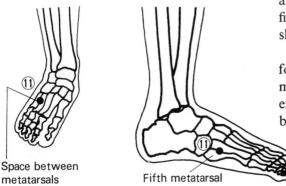

Space between metatarsals

Fifth metatarsal

The "number elevens" help balance the yang (posterior) Regulator and the Belt Channels. They influence the ankles, feet, and lower legs, and were also traditionally used for headaches, rheumatism, perspiration problems, and excessive bodily water weight.

⑫ (B 62)
This point is located just below the outer ankle-bone (outer malleolus) and may be tender upon pressure. Its position is similar to that of number nine.

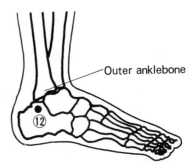

Outer anklebone

The "number twelves" help balance the yang Bridge Channel and can thus be used for insomnia, as one of their names "Calm Sleep" implies. They help release the feet and knees, and were also traditionally used for headaches, hypertension (high blood pressure), and pain control. They also help to release the lower back points.

⑬ (GB 34)
This point is found below the head, or top, of the fibula (the slender bone you will feel along the outside of the lower leg). To find it, go just below the protrusion you will feel at the top of the fibula, and between the fibula and tibia. Hold the point with pressure slightly towards the inner edge of the fibula.

The "number thirteens" are special points for the muscles and thus can be used for any muscle conditions, including soreness after exercise. They are very helpful for any yang body conditions. These points help release

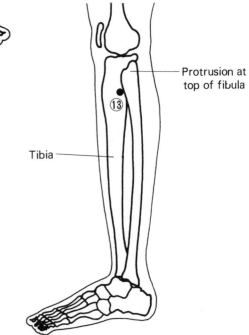

Protrusion at top of fibula

Tibia

the knees and legs, and were also traditionally used for headaches, abdominal problems, constipation, lower back tension, and
fear or extreme fright.

⑭ (GB 31)

This point is located just behind the thigh-
bone (femur) and about halfway between the
top of the femur and the knee. If you stand
up with your hands hanging at your sides,
palms against the thighs (see illustration at
right), this point will be located under the
middle fingertip on the outside of the thigh.
It may be quite sensitive to pressure.

The "number fourteens" help release the
outer thighs, knees, legs, and hip joints.
These points generally facilitate the release of
points on the back of the body (along the
yang parts of the Strange Flow routes) and
may be used for helping to clear physical or
emotional toxicity. They were also traditionally used for lower back problems and weakness of the legs.

⑮ (B 48)

This point is found just outside of the top of
the sacrum, in the "dimples" of the buttocks.
Follow the top of the pelvic bone (iliac crest)
from the outside of the hips to the place
where it meets the sacrum (sacroiliac joint).
To find the point, go about two fingers' width
outside of this meeting place. This will often
be a point of muscle tension and soreness
upon pressure. (It is more difficult to find
this point when the person is standing up, as
the muscles of the pelvic region, especially the
gluteus maximus, are very large. When the
person is lying down, these muscles will be
relaxed and finding the point will be easier.)

The "number fifteens" are associated with
the bladder. They are important points for
pelvic release and were also traditionally
used for abdominal problems, constipation,
hemorrhoids, and prostate or urinary problems.

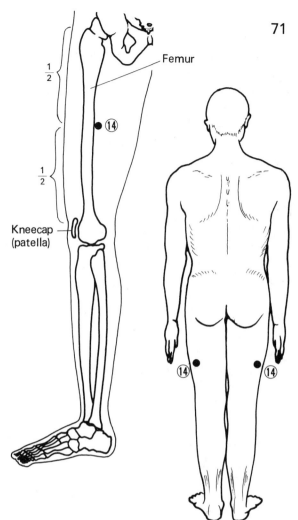

(Location point below middle fingertip)

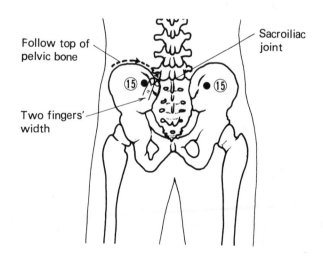

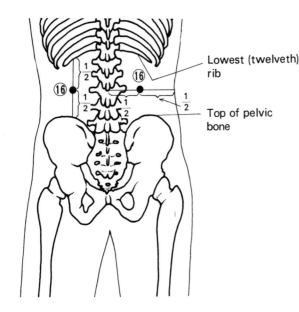

Lowest (twelveth) rib

Top of pelvic bone

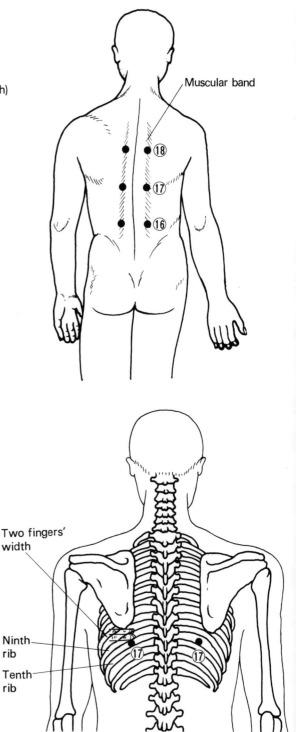

Muscular band

Two fingers' width

Ninth rib

Tenth rib

⑯ (B 47)

This point and the following two points are located on a long muscular band which can be felt along the entire back. Starting at the shoulders, between the scapula (shoulder blade) and spine, trace this band all the way down the back to the lumbar area.[1]

To find the number 16, draw a line from the lowest rib down to the top of the pelvic bone, and then divide this line in half. The point will be located at this level and about halfway between the sides of the body and the center of the spine. It is outside of the junction between the second and third lumbar vertebrae.

The "number sixteens" are associated with the kidneys. They strengthen the lower abdomen and are a central point for lower back release. They were also traditionally used for abdominal problems, appetite balance, all genital problems, and prostate or urinary problems. These points are used to strengthen the whole body.

⑰ (B 42)

This point is located between the ninth and tenth ribs and on the muscular band described above. Find the bottom of the scapu-

[1]You are feeling the deep muscle structure of the back— the "long" or longissimus muscle which lies under the superficial thoraco-lumbar fascia (♯16), latissimus dorsi muscle (♯17), and trapezius muscle (♯18).

la: if necessary, have the person rotate his shoulder so that you can feel the shoulder blade more easily. The point is located about two fingers' width below the bottom of the scapula and about halfway between its inner edge and the spine.

The "number seventeens" are associated with the liver. They help release the back, and they influence the diaphragm. These points were also traditionally used for fullness in the chest, poor digestion, and fainting.

⑱ (B 38)

This point is located between the fourth and fifth ribs. To find it, draw a line along the inside of the shoulder-blade (scapula), then divide this line in half from top to bottom. The point will be found at this level and halfway between the inner edge of the scapula and the spine. Often a knot of muscular tension like a marble will be felt at this point. If the band of muscle tension is continuous from the nineteens area through the eighteens to the seventeens, this point can usually be recognized by its sensitivity to pressure.

The "number eighteens" are associated with the circulation, and influence the respiration and the lungs. Because they strengthen the entire body, they were traditionally used for chronic conditions. They help release the upper back and facilitate shoulder, neck, and arm release. These points were also traditionally used for difficult breathing, coughing, hyperacidity, and tiredness.

⑲ (TW 15)

This point is located in a little hollow just above the top of the shoulder blade (scapula). It may be sensitive or tense, feeling like a marble or wiry band.

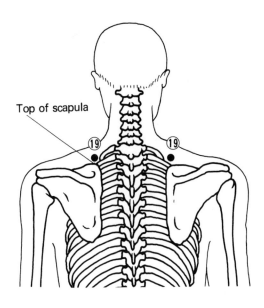

Top of scapula

The "number nineteens" (and the area around them) influence the body's resistance to "external evils," and were traditionally used to reduce fever and to open the perspiration. They help release the shoulders and scapulae, and facilitate release of the neck and arms. They were also traditionally used for hypertension and nervous tension.

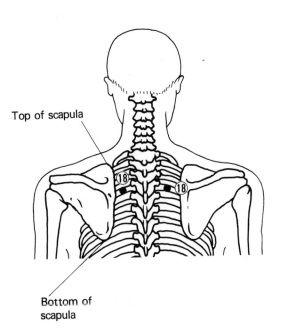

Top of scapula

Bottom of scapula

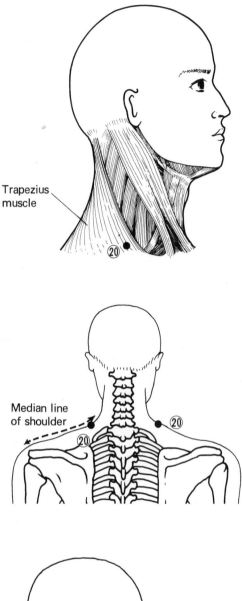

Trapezius muscle

Median line of shoulder

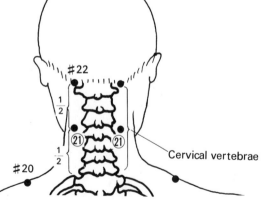

#22

#21

#20

Cervical vertebrae

⓴ (GB 21)

This point is located on the trapezius muscle at the base of the neck, where the neck begins to curve upward from the shoulder. It is found on the median line of the shoulder, about halfway between the front and back of the body. It is easy to recognize this point because it is usually very tense, like a marble or golf ball, and sore upon pressure.

The "number twenties" act like barometers of personal and cultural tension. When someone feels "uptight," usually these points are very tense, often actually pulling the shoulders up so that they are higher than is normal. Thus the area is literally "up" and "tight." These points help release neck and shoulder tension, as well as emotional feelings such as irritability and inability to cope.

They are also associated with the sexual organs and therefore should not be held with too much pressure nor worked on too vigorously on a pregnant woman. (But, for that matter, neither should any point.) These points were also traditionally used to help release headache, nervous conditions, tiredness, and throat problems. Their release is very important for the free passage of the Strange Flows up the neck and through the head.

㉑ (extra point)

This point is located about halfway between the top of the neck (where number 22 is located) and the base of the neck (where number 20 is located). It is found outside of the junction between the third and fourth cervical vertebrae, and about two fingers' width out from the center of the spine. Try to find the area of greatest tension, but be sure not to apply pressure too close to or on the spine. This point is not one of the 361 traditional acu-points, but is one of hundreds of extra, special points that have been discovered throughout the history of acupuncture and acupressure.

The area of the "number twenty-ones" is very important to the entire body, as most of the organ meridians or their branches, as well as the Regulator and Bridge Channels, flow through this narrow region. The particular point shown on the diagram helps release the neck, shoulder, and arm, and was also traditionally used for throat and voice problems and headaches.

㉒ (GB 20)

This point is located just below the base of the skull (the occipital bone), in a little hollow between the two muscle bands you will feel there (sternocleidomastoid and trapezius muscles). It is outside of the spinal column and will often be sensitive to pressure.

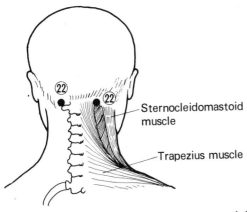

The "number twenty-twos" are especially important to the Regulator and Bridge Channels; indeed, their importance to the entire body cannot be overemphasized. These points influence the eyes, ears, nose, mouth, and brain. They help release neck and head tensions and strongly affect the consciousness; they were also traditionally used for colds and flus, dizziness, headaches, insomnia, and nervous problems.

㉓ (SI 10)

This point is located on the back of the shoulder just below the joint between the arm and shoulder. Follow the upper arm

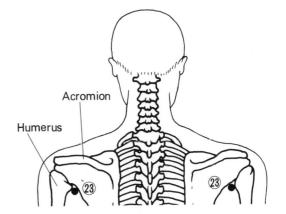

bone (humerus) up the back of the arm until you find a little hollow below the crest of the shoulder blade (acromion). The point may be sore upon pressure, and you may feel a band or knot of tight muscles.

The "number twenty-threes" influence the entire shoulder, scapula, and neck region, and facilitate the release of the major points in these areas. They were also traditionally used for hypertension (high blood pressure).

㉔ (LI 14)

This point is located just below the bulging muscle of the upper arm (deltoid). To find it, draw a line from the shoulder to the elbow, then divide that line by three. The point will be about 1/3 of the way down the arm, and in the middle of the arm from front to back.

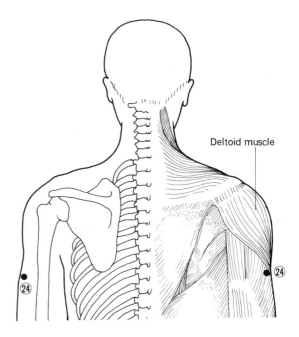

The "number twenty-fours" influence the arms and the shoulders, and facilitate release of the neck. They influence the large intestines and were also traditionally used for throat and teeth problems.

25 (LI 11)

This point is located in front of the elbow joint. To find it, the elbow must be bent until the crease at the inside of the elbow becomes clearly visible. The point is located just below the outer edge of the crease, and may be sensitive to pressure.

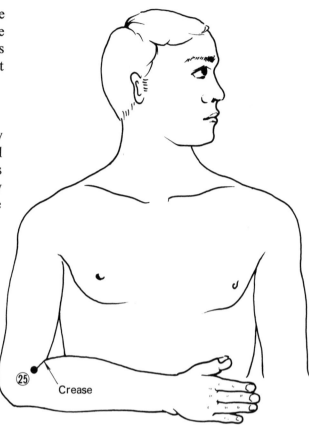

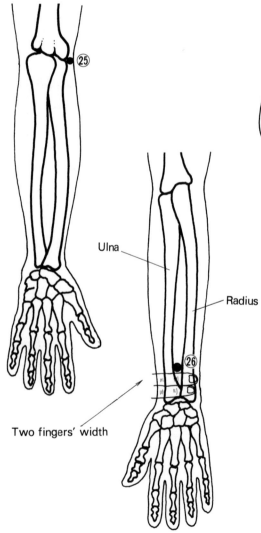

The "number twenty-fives" influence the arms and the elbows, and are said to stimulate the production of antibodies. They were also traditionally used for fever, hypertension (high blood pressure), constipation, and skin problems, as well as depression.

26 (TW 5)

This point is located above the wrist on the outside of the arm. It is found between the two bones of the lower arm (the radius and ulna) and about two fingers' width above the wrist.

The "number twenty-sixes" help balance the yang Regulator and the Belt Channels. They influence the arms, elbows, wrists, and fingers. These points were also traditionally used for colds and flus, headaches, rheumatism, and fear.

27 (P 6)

This point is found above the wrist on the inner arm, in a position similar to that of number 26. It is found about two fingers' width above the crease of the wrist and between the two bones of the forearm (radius and ulna) on the palm-side of the arm.

The "number twenty-sevens" help balance the yin Regulator and the Penetrating Channels, and are general pain points. They help release the arms, underarms, and elbows, and were also traditionally used for difficult breathing, dizziness, and nausea.

28 (P 3)

This point is located on the crease of the inner elbow region. Bend your arm slightly in order to see this crease and to feel the tendon in the middle of the crease. The point is located on the crease at the ulnar side of the tendon (of the biceps brachii muscle).

The "number twenty-eights" help release the arms, elbows, and shoulders. They were also traditionally used for cardiac and lung problems, feelings of dryness in the mouth and thirst, and vomiting.

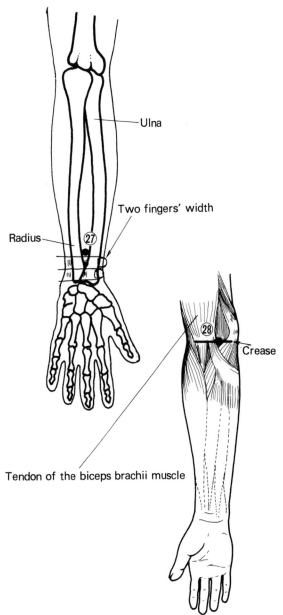

Ulna

Two fingers' width

Radius

27

Crease

28

Tendon of the biceps brachii muscle

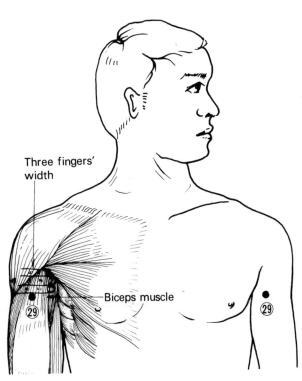

Three fingers' width

Biceps muscle

29

29

29 (P 2)

This point is located on the inner surface of the upper arm, within the biceps muscle. Its position is similar to that of number 24 on the outside of the arm. To find this point, place your index finger at the top of the armpit. You will find a little hollow below your ring fingertip, which will probably be sensitive to pressure.

The "number twenty-nines" help release the inside of the arms, and facilitate release of the upper back. They were also traditionally used for lung problems, fear of wind and cold, and palpitations from fear.

㉚ (Lu 1)

This point is located on the outside of the upper chest. It is found below the collarbone (clavicle) and just outside the rib-cage at a level about one finger's width above the underarm. It is outside of the third rib and will frequently be very blocked and tense.

The "number thirties" are associated with the lungs and help to free the breathing and release the chest and shoulders. When these points are very blocked, the person is usually feeling grief or oppression, or generally holding onto emotions. The number thirties were also traditionally used for coughing, skin problems, and tonsil problems. Their release encourages a relaxed and optimistic spirit.

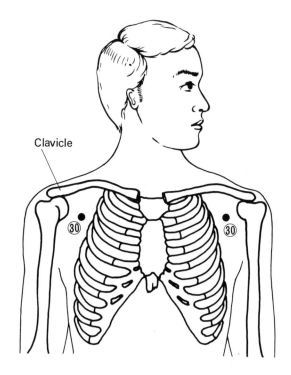

Clavicle

The more accurately you can feel and find each point, the more effective and efficient your acupressure treatments will be. However, it is not necessary to find and hold every point perfectly in order to give a very pleasant and relaxing Jin Shin Do treatment. Even beginners will be amazed at their innate skill in this simple effective art. As long as you look for the tense or sensitive spot in the area described, direct compassion to the other person, and concentrate on channeling and releasing ki, you will be good at Jin Shin Do right away!

7. THE TREATMENT TOUCH

There are many different ways of stimulating the points in acupressure treatments, but the most basic one is also the most important and effective. That method is simply holding the points. In this way you can contact the ki most strongly, release ki blockage most thoroughly, and channel the ki through the eight Strange Flows most effectively.

The points can be held with either your fingertips or your thumbs, and in some situations with the entire palm of your hand. Your choice of which to use will be guided by your own preferences and by the most convenient position for holding each point. Since the index and middle fingers tend to be the most sensitive, you may wish to use these when first locating points. Especially on areas of great tension, you may also use two or three fingertips together, giving stability to the main finger that is holding the point.

Although the method of direct finger pressure is a simple one, it is also capable of almost infinite development, for its subtleties are many. Perhaps the most frequent—and important—question is: "How much pressure should I use?" In this, we can be guided by two very basic Taoist principles: "the Middle Way" and "wei-wu-wei."

The Middle Way

In the amount of pressure used, neither the extreme of force nor the extreme of epidermal touch is as effective as the Middle Way of gentle but firm pressure. If a great amount of force is used so that excessive soreness or pain is felt at the points, not only will people not like to receive treatments from you, but

you are in fact by that very force blocking the ki flow rather than releasing and directing its flow. Additionally, the muscular tension that excess force creates in your own shoulders and arms can distort your own body posture, as well as prevent you from channeling ki through your hands and fingertips effectively. Because of this, and because the person usually tightens up in an automatic response to the pain, it will actually be more difficult to release the point!

The other extreme, a touch so light that it can barely be felt, not only may feel irritating to many people, but also will be ineffective for releasing points of great tension. At these points—the "beaver dams" of our earlier analogy—excess ki is trapped in tense muscles and has become stagnant, or too yin.

To understand the importance of releasing these points of ki blockage and muscular armoring, it may be helpful to look briefly at the development of chronic tension. Because a muscle is tight or tense, the circulation of blood and ki through it is impeded and "fatigue toxins" (the by-products of muscle work) build up. These cause the muscles to tense further, and eventually the fascial tissues (which surround muscles and enable their smooth movement) begin to adhere together. These "fascial adhesions" create larger and larger, harder and harder masses of muscle tension, which build up larger and larger blocks of stagnated ki.

"Man when living is soft and tender;
When dead he is hard and rough.
All animals and plants when living are
tender and fragile;

When dead they become withered and dry.
Therefore it is said:
The hard and tough are parts of death;
The soft and tender are parts of life.
This is the reason why the soldiers when
they are too tough cannot carry the day;
The tree when it is too tough will break.
The position of the strong and great is
low,
And the position of the weak and tender
is high."[1]

Almost everyone has many tense, hard, and blocked points. If we only use an epidermal touch, this will release the person's ki flow to some degree and this flow will itself begin to carry some of the stagnant ki away. However, unless the treater's channeling of ki is very strong, the core of tension will usually have been little reduced, and may soon resume its habitual pattern of impeding the ki flow.

It is necessary to release the muscle tension or armoring of the body, because this armoring with its content of past experiences prevents us from living in the here-and-now, from really being free. It is also necessary to release, direct, and balance the ki flow—so that the body can maintain a released state and resume its normal function of balancing itself, and also so that tension release can be easier and gentler. Although both the extremes of very deep and of epidermal touch have their uses, generally the "middle way" works best.

> *"In ruling men and in serving Heaven, the*
> *Sage uses only moderation.*
> *By moderation alone he is able to have*
> *conformed early (to Tao).*
> *This early conformity is called intensive*
> *accumulation of virtue.*
> *With this intensive accumulation of*
> *virtue, there is nothing he cannot*
> *overcome."*[2]

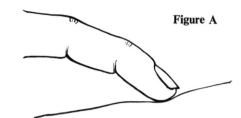

Figure A

At points of little or no tension or armoring, use a lighter touch and concentrate on feeling the ki.

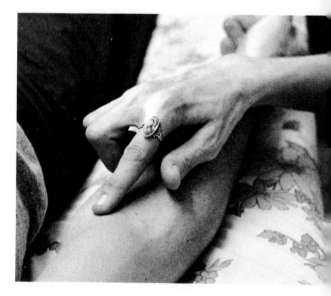

What is the middle way of finger pressure? At points where there is little or no muscular tension, apply firm but gentle pressure just until you feel that you are contacting the ki. You may use the pad of the finger rather than the tip. (See Figure A.) At points which feel tense, use just enough pressure to be onto the tension, so that you feel the hardness of the muscle at your fingertips. (See Figure B.)

To hold points on more yin areas, such as the chest, abdomen, or forehead, just let the weight of your arm sink onto the point. (See Figure C.) On more yang, muscular areas,

---

[1] *Tao Teh Ching*, from Chapter LXXVI.
[2] *Ibid.*, from Chapter LIX.

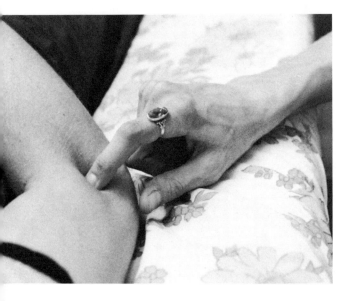

Figure B

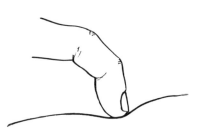

At points of muscular tension or armoring, gradually apply pressure until you are onto the tension.

Figure C

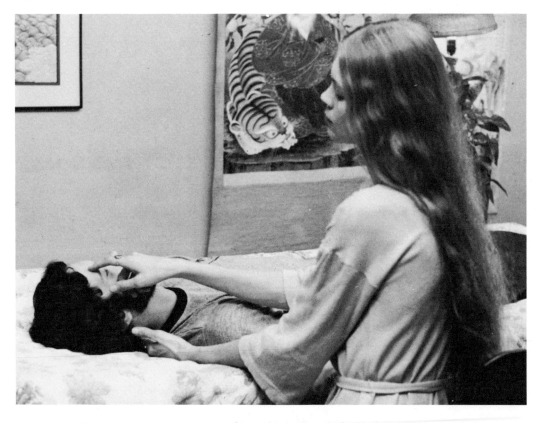

The right hand is holding point #1. Since this is on a yin body area and is not a point of great muscular tension, it is held with just the weight of the arm sinking onto the point.

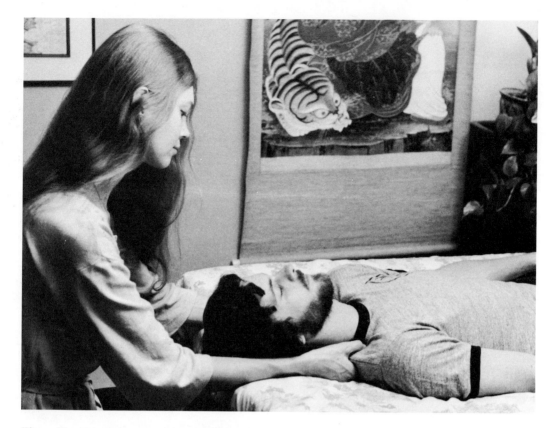

Figure D   Both hands are holding point # 20. Since this is on a yang, muscular area, and is often a point of tension, it is held with firm but not excessively strong pressure. With the thumbs on the # 20s, the treater here is leaning her body weight slightly into the points, so that muscular force is not required.

Figure E
The left hand is holding point # 15. Since this is a back point, the hand is in the position described at the right in order to make use of the person's body weight in holding the point with firm pressure.

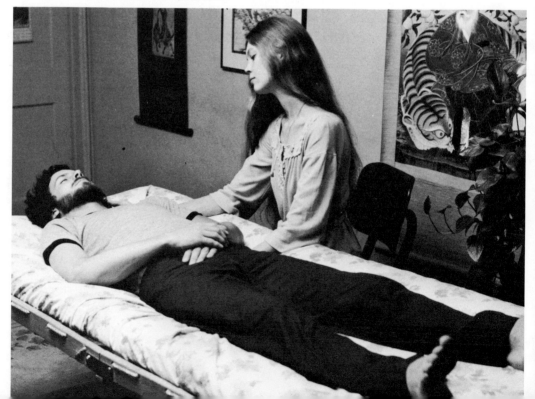

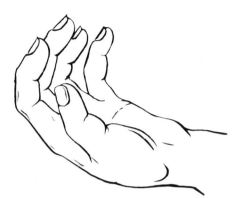

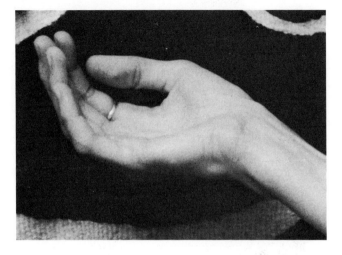

The hand is cupped as though holding a child's ball for working on back points. The fingertips are onto the point so that the person's body weight rests on the fingertips. The hand should be fairly relaxed.

apply firm but not forceful pressure, leaning into the point slightly with your body weight. (See Figure D.) For the back area (yang), a simple technique can be used to give the right amount of pressure. The person is usually lying on his or her back throughout the Jin Shin Do acupressure session. Slide your hand under the person's back, then curl your fingers upward as though to hold a child's ball. The weight of the person's body on your fingertips will generally be sufficient pressure. (See Figure E.)

To hold any point, apply the pressure gradually, letting the fingers sink slowly into the body until the tension is felt or, if there is little tension, enough to feel the ki flow. Do not apply pressure so deeply or strongly that the person is in pain, or so that you yourself are working too hard muscularly.

Giving a Jin Shin Do acupressure treatment should be good for you, as well as for the recipient. Following the middle way—applying just enough pressure to be onto the tension or to feel the ki flow—will enable you to do acupressure without putting stress on your own system. It also enables you to release the acu-points efficiently and peacefully,

facilitating the channeling of ki directly into the blocked area, and quickening the directing of stagnated ki out of that area.

For the recipient, the sensations of the touch are pleasant, so that there is little resistance. He or she is working with you, rather than consciously or sub-consciously against you. Therefore, "there is nothing that cannot (be) overcome." As the tension releases, your fingertips may follow the tension, sinking further into the body. It is rather like asking the body, "wouldn't you really like to release this?" rather than demanding or trying to force the letting go process. The peaceful yet deep release of ki that results from this approach is the real power and magic of Jin Shin Do.

Wei-wu-wei—The Relaxed Way of Doing

Releasing the ki flow in this way also follows the principle of wei-wu-wei. John Blofeld explains this principle clearly and practically: "Underlying all this is the great Taoist principle of not acting except in response to imperative need. When something has to be done, the wise man steps forward without fuss and deals with it as effectively as possible, but no sooner is the result ensured than he slips away to be free of unnecessary involvement. The true meaning of 'wei-wu-wei' is not 'doing by not doing'[1] but acting in a manner that entails the least involvement and proceeds from the inner stillness of the heart.'"[2]

Concentrating on the ki flow and on the release of blocked ki is "wei-wu-wei." It entails the least physical involvement. It proceeds from a compassionate Shin (Spirit, residing in the heart). It is the most direct way of releasing body-mind tensions, because it works harmoniously with the natural body forces and desires. And it is one of the most effective ways of increasing the absorption and use of ki. The deep state of relaxation and energy awareness that results is one in which the body is best able to regulate and balance itself.

Following the principle of wei-wu-wei, when we attain the desired release, we slip away from the point. Just as we applied pressure gradually, so we also gradually release the pressure, coming off the point slowly. Knowing how much each point should release in a treatment session requires experience. But you can look for three basic indication of sufficient release:

1) a feeling of actual softening in the muscles around the point;
2) a decrease or release of sensitivity or soreness at the point;
3) a feeling of strong, orderly, and regular pulsation at the point.

Each point should be held for at least thirty seconds; one minute is an average holding time. Very tense and armored points may be held longer—for perhaps two minutes or more.

The third indication, the pulsation, is not the blood pulse and is not merely the pulsation of your own fingertips. Of course, you may feel a pulsation in your fingertips as you hold points, especially at first when this new use of your fingers is increasing the circulation in them. However, the pulsation in your fingertips is a fairly constant one, whereas the pulsation that will be felt at the points is always changing. If the point is very blocked, at first you may not feel any pulsation; as the blocked ki releases, you will feel a pulsation beginning and then gradually becoming stronger and more orderly. Feeling this ki pulsation at the acu-points is an experience in itself!

It is normal to be somewhat skeptical of things like ki pulsation, or of the possibilities of ourselves feeling and experiencing these things. After all, they have not usually been a part of our western cultural training. One student, a nurse, while being receptive to learning about oriental health philosophies and practices, also typified this general skepticism or reservation, wondering whether the pulsation described was not simply that of the blood. Then one night she came to class exclaiming, "I'm so excited! I just felt the pulse—and it's not the blood!" In this, as in all other discoveries, be patient with yourself. If you do not feel this third indication at first, just look for the tension release, or just hold the points for the time described.

Wei-wu-wei also means using a minimum of points and treatment patterns to affect the result. It is not necessary or desirable to stimulate every acupressure point on the body, or even all of the thirty main Jin Shin Do points. Thus the Jin Shin Do treatment patterns have been designed on the basis of efficiency, using a limited number of remarkable points within formulae general enough to be used on most people.

[1]Common definition of wei-wu-wei.
[2]*The Secret and the sublime: Taoist Mysteries and Magic*, by John Blofeld, Dutton, 1973, page 163.

Treatment Position

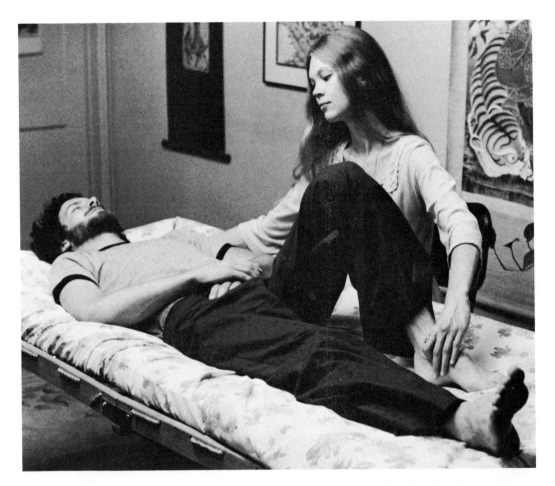

Figure F The recipient of the treatment is lying on her back on a cot. The left hand is over the hara region, so that the palm is resting on the belly. The right hand is placed over the left hand. This position allows the treater to hold any of the Jin Shin Do points, and if desired to direct the recipient in hara breathing, without asking the recipient to change positions.

The person to be treated usually lies down on his or her back and maintains that position throughout the Jin Shin Do acupressure treatment. The recipient's hands may be folded over the hara region, with the right hand on top of the left. (See Figure F.) Or they may remain at the sides of the body if that is more comfortable.

Since your hands must move under the person's body in order to hold the points on the back as described earlier, it is best to have the recipient lie on a cot with a fairly thick foam cushion on top (covered with a sheet). In this way, movement under the body will be quite easy, although you may ask the person to raise his or her buttocks or back slightly if you have trouble sliding underneath these areas at first, or if the person is very muscular or overweight.

You may use a low cot and sit in tradition-

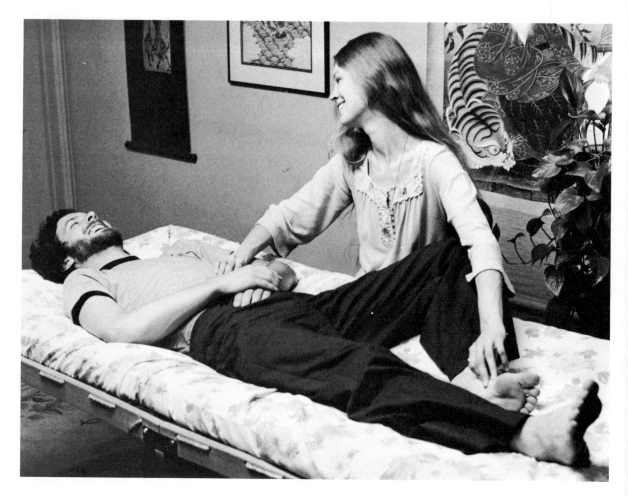

Figure G

al Japanese, cross-legged, or other positions beside the cot. Or you may use a regular massage table (again, with foam cushion and covering sheet) or a special Jin Shin table, and sit on a chair or stool beside the table. This is usually the most comfortable way to give a treatment, especially if you eventually give two or more treatments in a row. If cots or tables are not available, a bed may be used. The person's head should be at the foot of the bed, as sometimes it is necessary to work on the neck points while sitting at the head of the person. A couch may also be used, as long as the armrests are not too high. The recipient may just lie on a mat on the floor, or even on the floor itself, but this is usually the least comfortable position for the treater.

Why does the person being treated remain on his back, rather than turning onto his stomach, while you work on his back? For two main reasons: 1) changing positions in this way would interrupt the recipient's relaxed meditative state, and 2) it is actually easier to work on the back, using direct pressure, when the person lies on his back.

If the person laid on his stomach, you would have to stand, sit, or kneel above him and then either apply pressure using the muscular force of your arm, or else use your body weight to lean into the point. Either way, a fair amount of exertion is required on your part. However, if the person instead lies on his back, and your fingertips are resting on the point as described earlier, the person's body weight will do the work for you.

If you cannot reach points on the feet and lower legs comfortably, you may bend the person's leg as in Figure G.

Your fingers may get a little tired at first; this is true whenever you begin to use them in new ways, be it massage, piano, guitar, typing, or whatever. If this occurs, simply do a shorter treatment until your finger strength increases, which it will do very quickly. And, again, be sure that you are not using excessive force. The person you are working on should be encouraged to give you feedback and to tell you if any point feels very sore. Your fingers should be just onto the tension —not boring through it!

Beginning to Do Acupressure Release

Jin Shin Do treatment sessions are usually close to one hour in length, though of course they may be shorter—forty-five, thirty, fifteen, or even five minutes can be very helpful. To start using the points and practicing the treatment touch, you may try some or all of the following short acupressure release patterns. These two-step releases

may be done on just the tensest side of the body, or else on both sides of the body. You can start by practicing any one of these patterns by itself. Or you can begin with the first pattern and do each one consecutively. To do every pattern shown below in this way will probably take about forty-five minutes, depending on how long you hold the points.

Lower Back and Abdomen

Step 1:
One hand holds point #16:

While the other hand holds point #5:

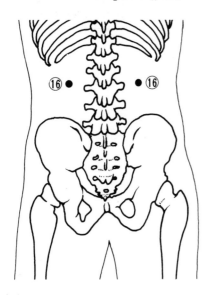

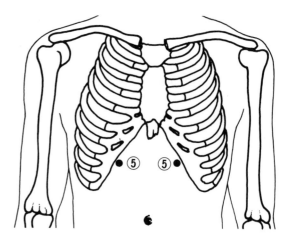

Step 2:
One hand remains on point #16.

While the other hand moves off point #5 and instead holds point #13.

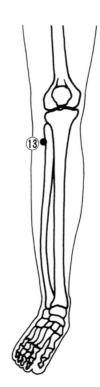

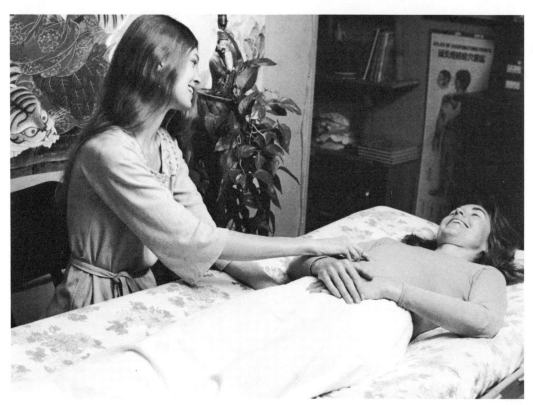

Step 1

Step 2

Lower Back and Abdomen Illustrated:

Step 1:
The treater is working on the right back. She is holding the ♯16 with her left hand. At the same time, she is holding the ♯5 on the same side of the body with her right hand. (To work on the left back, you will sit at the left side of the person. You will hold the ♯16 with your right hand, and the ♯5 with your left hand.)

Step 2:
The left hand remains on the ♯16, but the right hand has moved down to the ♯13. (When working on the left ♯16, it will be your left hand that moves to ♯13.)

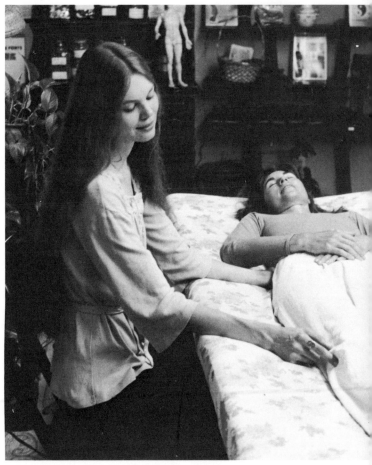

Neck and Face

Step 1:
  One hand holds point #21:

While the other hand holds point #1:

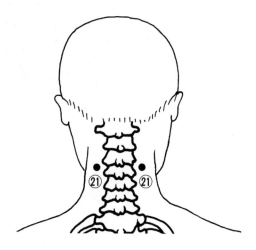

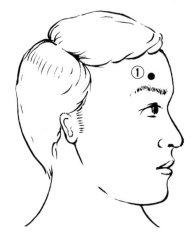

Step 2:
  One hand remains on point #21:

While the other hand moves off point #1 and instead holds point #2:

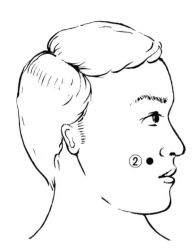

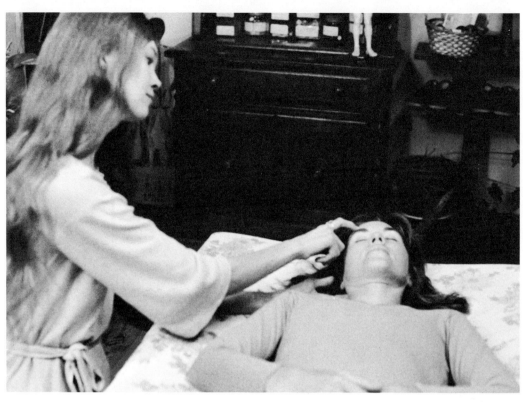

Neck and Face Illustrated:

Step 1:

The treater is working on the right neck. She is holding the #21 with her left hand. At the same time, she is holding the #1 on the same side of the body with her right hand. (To work on the left neck, you will sit at the left side of the person. You will hold the #21 with your right hand, and the #1 with your left hand.)

Step 2:

The left hand remains on the #21, but the right hand has moved down to the #2. (When working on the left #21, it will be your left hand that moves to #2.)

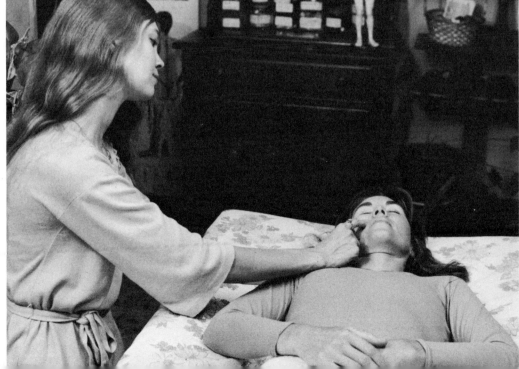

Shoulders

Step 1:
One hand holds point #20:

While the other hand holds point #26:

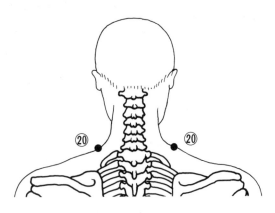

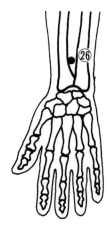

Step 2:
One hand moves off point #20 and instead holds point #19:

While the other hand remains on point #26.

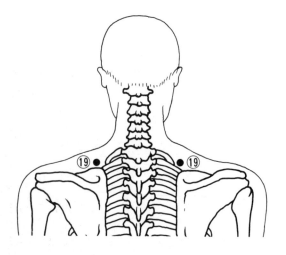

Shoulders Illustrated:

Step 1:
The treater is working on the right shoulder. She is holding the #20 with her left hand. (It may be easiest to hold this point with the thumb.) At the same time, she is holding the #26 on the same side of the body with her right hand. (To work on the left shoulder, you will sit at the left side of the person. You will hold the #20 with your right hand, and the #26 with your left hand.)

Step 2:
The left hand has moved down to the #19, but the right hand remains on the #26. (When working on the left #20, it will be your right hand that moves down to the #19.)

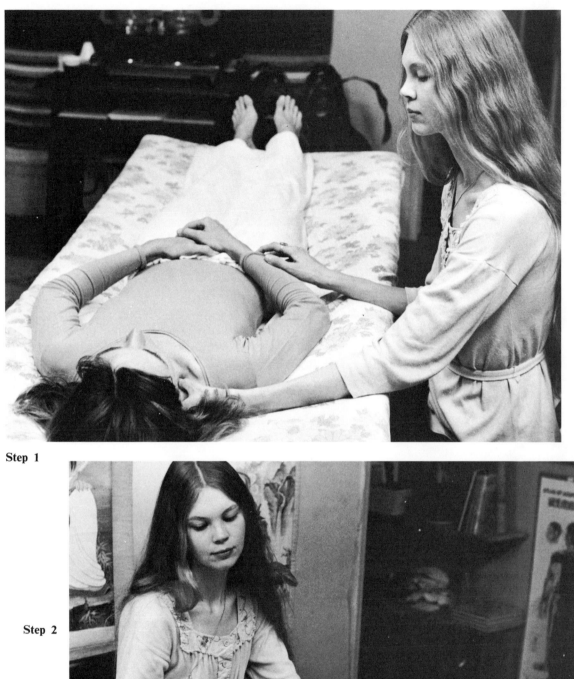

Step 1

Step 2

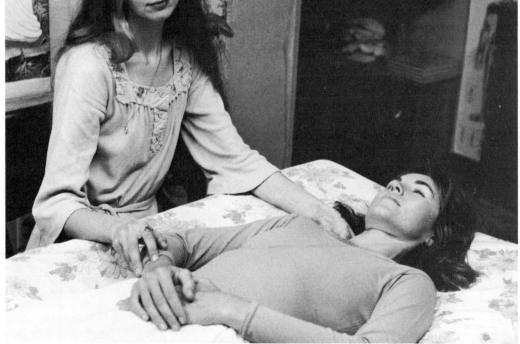

94

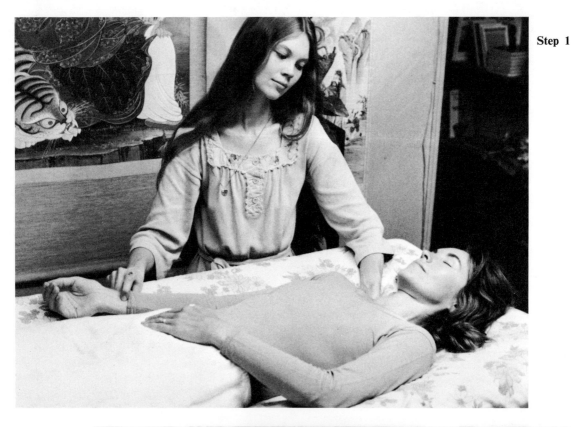

Step 1

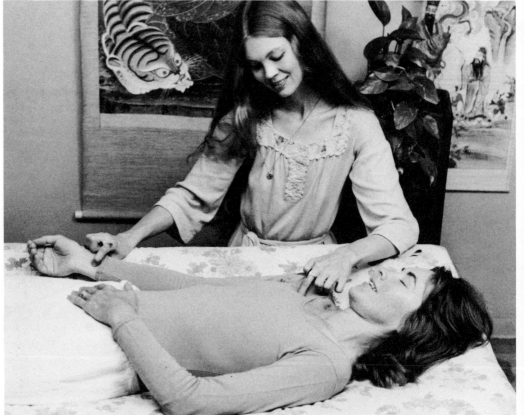

Step 2

Upper Back and Chest

Step 1:
One hand holds point #18:

While the other hand holds point #27:

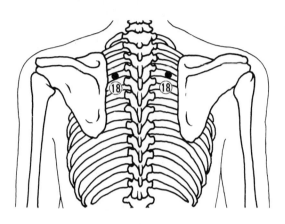

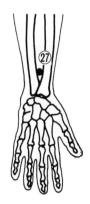

Step 2:
One hand moves off point #18 and instead holds point #30:

While the other hand remains on point #27.

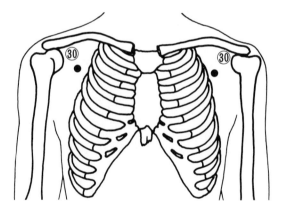

Upper Back and Chest Illustrated:

Step 1:
The treater is working on the right upper back and chest. She is holding point #18 with her left hand. (It may be easier to slide your hand down the back from the neck, as shown, rather than under the entire back.) At the same time, she is holding point #27 with her right hand. (To work on the left upper back and chest, you will sit on the left side of the person. You will hold the #18 with your right hand and the #27 with your left hand.)

Step 2:
The left hand has moved to the #30, but the right hand remains on the #27. (When working on the left #18, it will be your right hand that moves to the #30.)

Pelvic Area and Heels

Step 1:
One hand holds point #15:   While the other hand holds point #9:

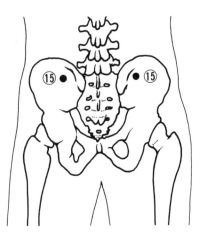

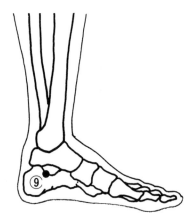

Step 2:
One hand remains on point #15:   While the other hand moves off point #9 and instead holds point #12.

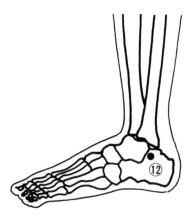

Pelvic Area and Heels Illustrated:

Step 1:
The treater is working on the right pelvic area. She is holding the #15 with her left hand. At the same time, she is holding the #9 on the same side of the body with her right hand. (To work on the left pelvic area, you will sit at the left side of the person. You will hold #15 with your right hand and #9 with your left hand.)

Step 2:
The left hand remains on the #15, but the right hand has moved to the #12. (When working on the left #15, it will be your left hand that moves to #12.)

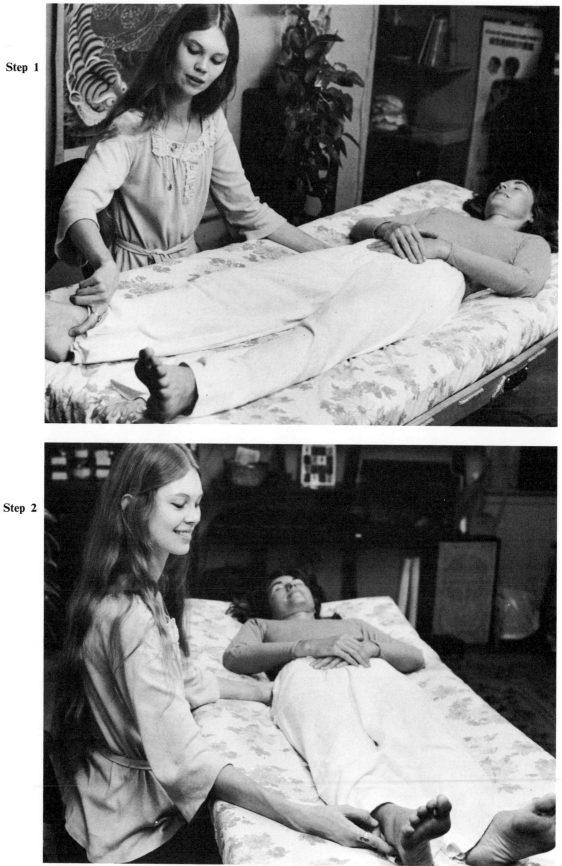

Basic Neck Release

The following five-step acupressure pattern is a very important one. This basic neck release, or a variation of it, is used at the end of almost every Jin Shin Do acupressure session. If you have done most or all of the above short patterns, then you have just given your first Jin Shin Do treatment! It would be a good idea to finish the treatment with this short release.

Step 1:
   Both hands hold the points #23:

Step 2:
   Both hands hold the points #19:

Step 3:
   Both hands hold the points #20:

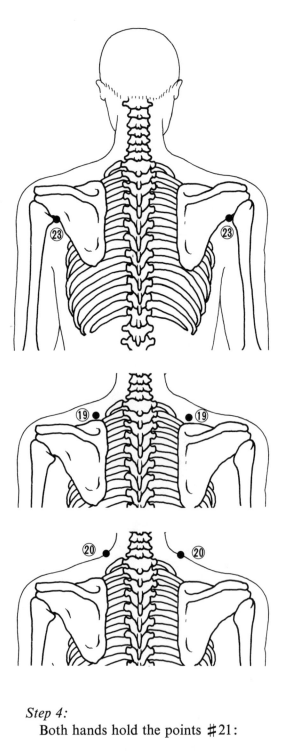

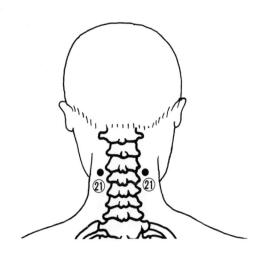

Step 4:
   Both hands hold the points #21:

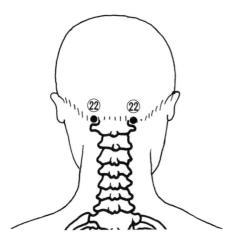

Step 5:
Both hands hold the points ♯22.

Basic Neck Release Illustrated:

Step 1

Step 1:
The treater is working on the ♯23s. With her fingertips under the outside of the shoulders, she is holding the left ♯23 with her left hand and the right ♯23 with her right hand. With her fingers curled and her fingertips on the points, the treater is using her body weight to lean into the points slightly.

Step 2

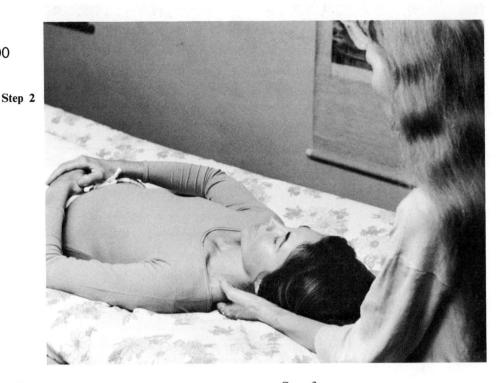

Step 2:

The treater is now working on the ♯19s. She is holding the left ♯19 with her left hand and the right ♯19 with her right hand. With the fingertips on the ♯19s, the thumbs can be in position to hold the ♯20s in the next step.

Step 3:

The treater next works on the ♯20s. With her hands in the position described above, she holds the left ♯20 with her left thumb and the right ♯20 with her right thumb. In this position, the treater can use her body weight to lean into the points slightly. (This is a suggested position; if it seems easier, the points may of course be held with the finger-tips.)

Step 3

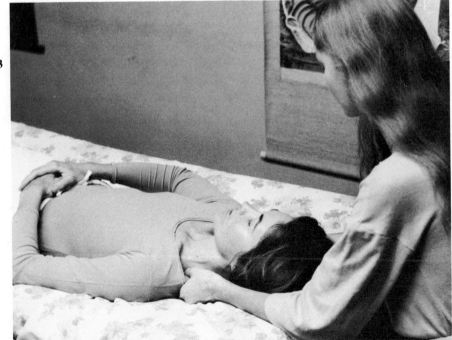

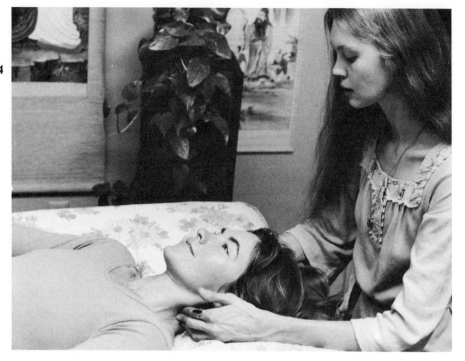

Step 4

Step 4:

The treater has moved up to the ♯21s. She is holding the left ♯21 with her left hand and the right ♯21 with her right hand. She will be looking for the tensest point in the area outside of the spine. The student should note that the ♯21 in this step and the ♯22 in the next step should be released at least as much as the ♯20s were in the preceding step.

Step 5:

Finally, the treater has moved up to the ♯22s. The left hand is holding the left ♯22, and the right hand is holding the right ♯22. The fingertips are used to hold these points. It is probably easiest to hold these points if the back of the head is cradled in the treater's hands, so that the person's head is resting on the treater's palms as shown below. Note that the treater is using her body weight to

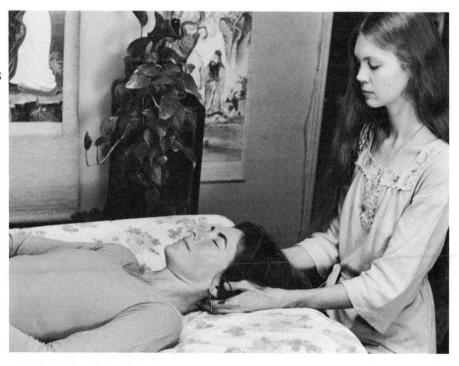

Step 5

lean back slightly, pulling the fingertips onto the base of the skull. The ♯22s are usually fairly easy to release after the points ♯23, 19, 20, and 21 have been released; however, their release is very important. Close your eyes while holding these points so that you can more easily feel and tune into them.

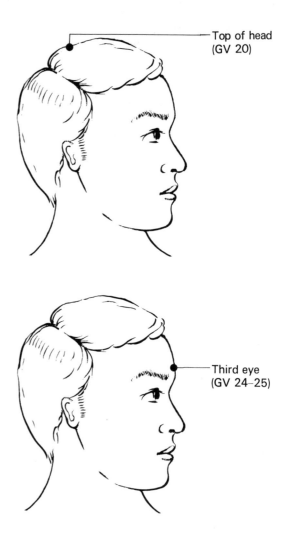

Top of head (GV 20)

Third eye (GV 24–25)

Short Centering Release

This one-step pattern may be used following the Basic Neck Release, or by itself.

Step 1:
    The right hand holds the point at the center top of the head:
    While the left hand holds the point between the eyebrows known as the "third eye":

Final Balancing Step

This one-step pattern may be used at the very end of a treatment session, after the Basic Neck Release and Short Centering Release.

Step 1:
    The right hand holds the point at the base of the sternum:

While the left hand holds both big toes:

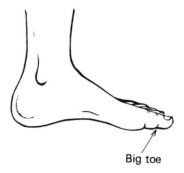

Big toe

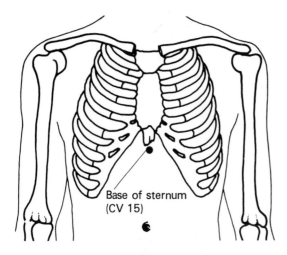

Base of sternum (CV 15)

Though there are several acu-points on the big toe, the main importance of holding it here is that the big toe is a cross-roads of several different energy flows.

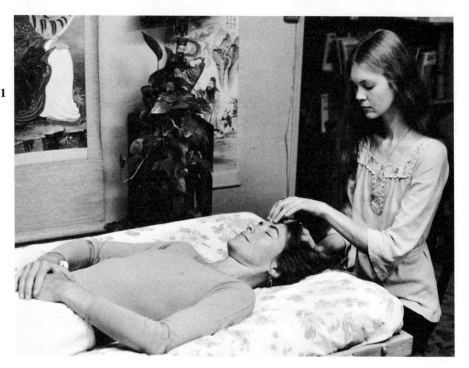

Short Centering Release Illustrated: ▲

Final Balancing Step Illustrated: ▼

Step 1:

The treater is holding the point at the top of the head with her right hand. (This point is located on the crown, where you will feel a little hollow.) With the fingertips of her left hand, she is holding the "third eye" gently. (This point is located between the eyebrows, in the center of the forehead.)

Step 1:

The treater is holding the point at the base of the sternum with the fingertips of her right hand. This point should be held gently. The palm may rest gently on the person's solar plexus region if you wish. With her left hand, the treater is holding both big toes, simply wrapping her hand around them. The treater has her eyes closed and is meditating on the general circulation of the ki up the back and down the front of the person.

Step 1

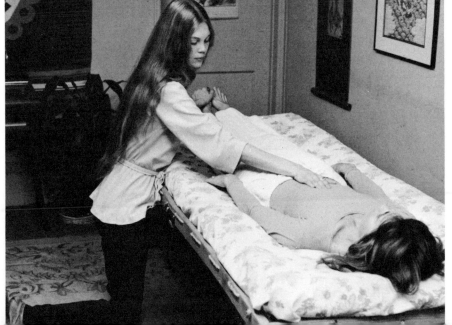

Self-Treatment

Any of the short acupressure patterns given in this chapter can also be done by yourself on yourself. You may choose one or two that seem appropriate, or else do the entire sequence. When working on yourself, just use gentle pressure. Tensing some of your muscles in order to release others is not an effective overall relaxing method!

Either sit on a chair or lie on the floor (or other firm surface) to do a self-treatment. To hold most of the points, just use gentle fingertip pressure. To hold points on the back, make your hand into a fist and place the knuckles against the point, then lean back in the chair (or relax on the floor, lying on your back) so that your body weight holds the point. When necessary, use opposite hands from those used above in working on others. Except for the Short Centering Release and the Final Balancing Step, your choice of hands can be based on convenience.

Holding the ♯21 and the ♯2 on yourself:

The subject is working on the right neck, holding the right ♯21 with his left hand, and the right ♯2 with his right hand. The position shown has the advantage of also stretching out the shoulders and upper chest. However, if you cannot keep your arm relaxed in this position, just let the left elbow hang down at the side of the body.

Holding the ♯18 and the ♯29 on yourself:

The ♯18 is perhaps the most difficult point to reach on yourself. If you cannot reach the ♯18 without straining, just reach as close to the point as possible at first. As you release your acu-points, you will gradually become more flexible.

The subject is working on his left upper back, holding his left ♯18 with his left hand,

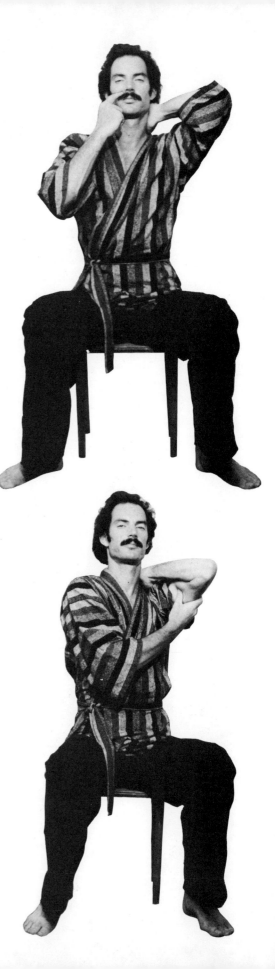

and the ♯29 with his right hand. Note that here opposite hands must be used from those previously illustrated for treatment on others.

Holding the ♯20s on yourself:

To hold points ♯19 or 20, hold the points with your fingertips. Then let your arms hang down so that the weight of your arms hold the points. The subject has the arms crossed so that the right hand holds the left ♯20, and the left hand holds the right ♯20. The hands need not be crossed; if it feels more comfortable to just hold the right point with the right hand and the left point with the left hand, do so.

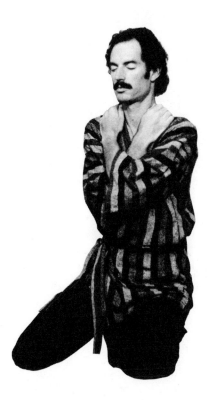

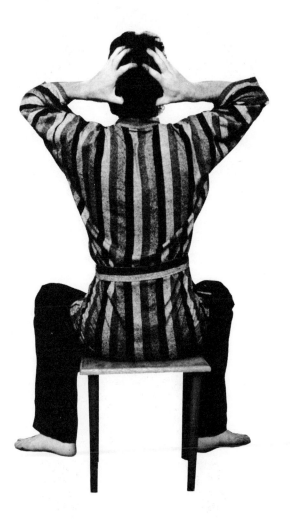

Holding the ♯22s on yourself:

With both palms on the back of the head, the subject is holding the ♯22s with the thumbs. This is an especially comfortable position if you are working on yourself while lying down on your back. You will then be cradling your head in your hands, and the weight of your head on your thumbs will hold the points with sufficient pressure. When doing a self-treatment sitting up, you may instead hold these points with your fingertips if you wish.

Doing the Short Centering Release on your-self:

The subject is holding the point at the top of the head with the right hand. Note that this point may be held by simply covering the top of the head with the palm of the hand. The subject is also holding the "third eye," with the left hand. Gentle fingertip pressure is used at this point. The eyes are closed so that the subject can better concentrate on the ki flow up the back and down the front of the body.

Even if you do not have a recipient at hand, you can practice the Jin Shin Do acupressure patterns just by working on yourself. Traditionally, the student of any oriental health art worked on himself or herself a great deal, either before or in addition to practicing on other persons. It was said that an acupuncturist, for example, should needle himself 1000 times before using needles on someone else. Since the gentle fingertip pressure technique of acupressure is completely safe to use, it is not necessary to practice on yourself before working on someone else. However, doing a self-treatment will be good for you, and it will also give you some idea of what the person you are treating is feeling, and of how the points feel.

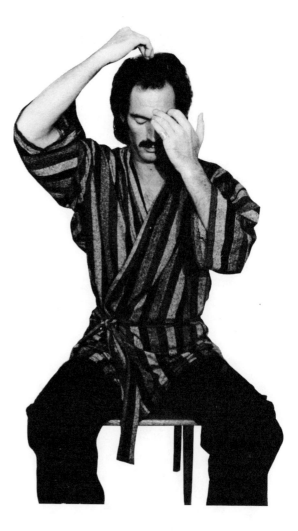

Simple Central Channel Release

Many students give themselves a simple Great Central Channel acupressure release in the morning before arising. The Great Central Channel, as we have seen, is the great sea of yin and yang, and the ruling energy channel of the entire body. Since it follows the spinal column up the back of the body and the median line down the front, its points are all unilateral, rather than bilateral like the thirty main Jin Shin Do points. These points will be easy to find from the diagrams below, and should be held with gentle fingertip pressure. This self-treatment is perhaps best done while lying on your back on a firm surface, and is especially effective if you do hara breathing at the same time.

This acupressure release pattern can also be done for someone else, either by itself or else in addition to some of the above short release patterns. In the latter case, you may begin the treatment session with this Central pattern, or else you may do this pattern before or after doing the Basic Neck Release.

Step 1:

The left hand holds the point just below the base of the sternum:

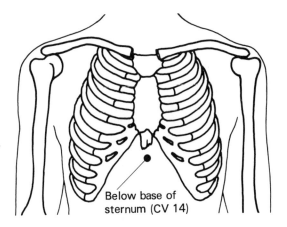

Below base of sternum (CV 14)

Step 2:

The left hand remains on the point just below the base of the sternum:

While the right hand holds the point at the top of the pubic bone (illustrated above).

Step 3:

The left hand still remains at the base of the sternum:

While the right hand moves to the point at the tip of the coccyx.

Step 4:

The left hand moves to the point located between the seventh cervical and first thoracic vertebrae (the two large vertebrae you will feel at the base of the neck):

While the right hand holds the hara (with the fingertips or with the entire palm).

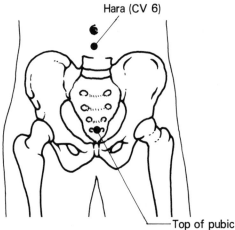

Hara (CV 6)

Top of pubic bone (CV 2)

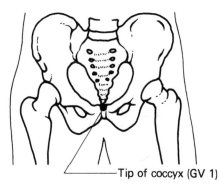

Tip of coccyx (GV 1)

While the right hand moves to the point located between the second and third lumbar vertebrae (inside of the ♯16s).

Between second and third lumbar vertebrae (Gv 4)

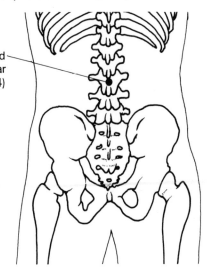

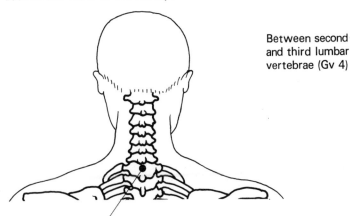

Between seventh cervical and first thoracic vertebrae (Gv 14)

Step 5:

The left hand moves to the point at the base of the skull:

While the right hand remains on the point between the second and third lumbar vertebrae.

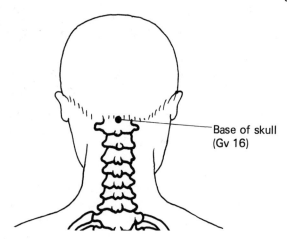

Base of skull
(Gv 16)

Step 6:

The left hand moves to the point between the eyebrows known as the "third eye":

While the right hand moves to the point at the top of the head:

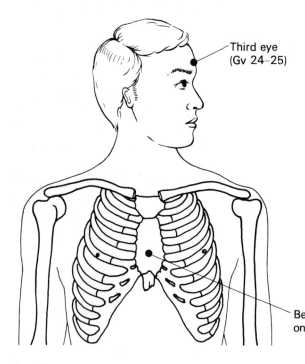

Third eye
(Gv 24–25)

Between nipples
on sternum (Cv 17)

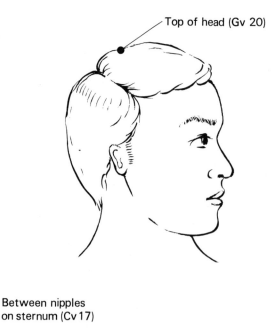

Top of head (Gv 20)

Step 7:

The left hand moves to the point between the nipples on the sternum (illustrated above):

While the right hand remains on the point at the top of the head.

8. HOW TO GIVE A JIN SHIN DO ACUPRESSURE TREATMENT

You have already learned the basic Jin Shin Do treatment method. Using this method, we will now learn to do acupressure patterns which release and balance each of the four pairs of Strange Flows, as well as patterns which work on various areas of the body more completely than the short patterns of the preceding chapter. We will continue to hold two points at the same time, one with the right hand and one with the left, as this is the most effective way of guiding the ki through the channels and meridians, and of releasing blocked or tense points.

A Release Shorthand

In order to present these longer Jin Shin Do acupressure patterns more easily, we will use a simple shorthand notation: "RH" indicates that the point is held with the right hand, and "LH" indicates that the point is held with the left hand. Following either of these notations there will be a dash and then a small letter "r" or "l." The "r" indicates that the point to be held will be located on the right side of the person's body, and the "l" indicates that it will be located on the left side of the body. Finally, the last indication on each line will be a number. This indicates the actual Jin Shin Do point to be held. You can refer to the charts next to each release

pattern to remind yourself of the point locations until you have the points memorized. The recipient will be lying on his or her back as described in the last chapter, and you will apply firm but gentle pressure at each point until the three indications—ki pulsation, tension release, and decrease of sensitivity —are noticed, or for an average of one to two minutes.

If there is a bracket around two lines of notation, this means that both hands move to the points indicated at the same time. If there is no bracket, just keep each hand on the point it is holding until there is an indication to move it. Remember that you will always have both hands holding points on the person's body.

For example, here is a pattern similar to the short "Neck and Face" release from the preceding chapter, written in this release shorthand:

Right flow— sit at right:	Left flow— sit at left:
⌠LH–r 21	⌠RH–l 21
⌡RH–r 1	⌡LH–l 1
RH–r 2	LH–l 2
LH–r 22	RH–l 22

Notice that the notations are given both for the "right flow" (the point and channel or meridian of ki flow on the right side of the body) and for the "left flow" (point and energy flow on the left side). To do the right side you are told to sit at the right side of the person. Since there is a bracket around the first two lines, you will place both the right and left hands on the points indicated at approximately the same time. Thus, your left hand will hold the person's right #21, while your right hand holds the person's right #1. The hands will stay this way until you feel a pulse at the right #1 (about thirty seconds to one minute). The #1 is not a point of great muscular tension, so feeling the ki pulsation is the most important indication of release here.

The third line in the above example indicates that the right hand moves to the person's right #2. Since the left hand is not told to do otherwise, it stays on the right #21. Hold the point #2 until you feel the ki pulsation and a relaxation of the area, and until any sensitivity felt upon pressure has decreased (about one to two minutes).

By this time, you should also be feeling a ki pulsation at the #21. The muscular tension or armoring at this point should be somewhat released, at least at the surface level, and the point should be less sensitive to pressure. If you do not feel that the #21 has released enough, just continue holding it with the #2 a little longer. Then the left hand is told to move the left #22. Since the right hand is not told to do otherwise, it stays on the right #2 (because that point helps to release the #22).

Since the #21 is held throughout most of this short pattern, it is the "base point" for this pattern. A "base point" is a point of great muscular tension and ki blockage which is held for several steps during a treatment pattern at least partially designed for its release.

The release patterns given in this chapter are longer than the above example, but as long as you remember to just leave either hand where it is until it is told to move, you will be able to decode them all quite easily.

Most people have more tension on one side of the body than on the other. In order to balance the body, we usually work mainly on the tightest side. For example, if the right side of the body is generally the tightest, you would probably do the "right flow" of whatever release pattern you chose. There are two exceptions to this general rule: 1) the Basic Neck Release is designed to work on both sides of the shoulders and neck, as the entire area is usually released with this pattern at the end of a treatment session; and 2) if both sides of the body are similar in tension, or if both sides are very tense, you may choose to work on both sides. In that case, you would do both the "right flow" and the "left flow" of whatever release pattern(s) you chose.

As you work with someone, giving him or her a series of acupressure treatments or perhaps continuous weekly sessions, you will eventually find yourself working on both sides of the body. If the right side is tenser than the left at first, you may first work mainly on it. After it releases, you may also wish to release the left side, which will probably also be somewhat tense and armored. The process of release is thus rather like peeling an onion—layer by layer, side by side.

Keep in mind the fact that you are not just working on tense body areas, however, you are working on acu-points and, primarily, on energy flows. This is the way acupressure works.

Treatment Format

In deciding how to combine several of the following release patterns within a treatment session (forty-five minutes to one hour), you may choose between three general treatment formats:

1) At first—both as you are beginning to treat and when a person is receiving his or her first treatment or two—it is a good idea to work on one of the four pairs of Strange Flows. (See pages 112–119.) These overall body balancing patterns will both release major points of tension and also balance the energy flows through which the body can regulate itself.

2) Or, you may first release one of the Strange Flow pairs, then also do a body area release to work further on the main ki blockages and imbalances.

3) Or, you may do only body area releases, choosing one, two, or three of these to work directly on the individual's primary tensions and ki blockages. (See pages 124–139.)

You may also add any of the short acupressure patterns given in the last chapter into any of the above treatment formats.

Always end the treatment session with the neck release and "end of treatment" patterns. (See pages 122–123.) Exceptions to this rule would be very short acupressure treatments, working on only a few points. Whenever the entire body is worked on and main tension points are released, ending the treatment with the Basic Neck Release or some variation of it is most important.

What is next? Do a treatment! The best way to begin is to just start treating, rather than trying to read through the treatment patterns intellectually. Have a friend lie down, and do a treatment for him or her. Even if you are a complete beginner at finger pressure arts, as long as you attempt to follow the general outlines already given, visualize channeling ki, and most importantly treat with compassion, your friend will enjoy the experience of your very first complete Jin Shin Do treatment—and so will you!

As long as you follow the release patterns as given and do not apply too much pressure, your first treatment will be successful and beneficial. Remember to encourage feedback from the recipient occasionally throughout the treatment session, to be sure that you are using the middle way of finger pressure, and also to help the recipient become more aware of his or her own condition. Sometimes people will not tell you whether you are holding a point too strongly or too lightly unless you ask. So don't be afraid to ask, "How does this feel?" or "Is this point sensitive?"

If a friend is not immediately available, work on yourself, following the suggestions given in the last chapter for self-treatment. Skip points you cannot comfortably reach or use opposite hands if necessary, excepting on points of the Great Central Channel.

Releasing the Strange Flows

Of course, all Jin Shin Do treatment patterns help to release and balance the eight Strange Flows, because the thirty main points are all Strange Flow points. However, sometimes you will wish to concentrate on releasing and balancing one pair of Strange Flows in particular. The following four release patterns are designed for that purpose, and help to release each of the four pairs of Strange Flows quite thoroughly. Thus, they enable the body to better regulate itself. If you do no other Jin Shin Do treatment patterns, you will be able to help people very much just with the use of these.

Because each of the following four release patterns is designed to regulate the entire pathway of a Strange Flows pair, they are a little longer than the average Jin Shin Do release pattern. However, each can comfortably be done within twenty–thirty minutes. You may refer to the diagrams and discussions in chapter 5 for help in choosing the

most effective of these four treatment patterns for each individual. Or you may just
choose any one and begin!

Great Regulator Channel

This treatment pattern is designed to release
and balance the Great Regulator Channel
in general (see pages 56–57). It is a very good
general release for the entire body. It is also
a good release for the neck and shoulders,
as its base points are ♯ 21, 19, and 23.

Regulator Release:

Right flow— sit at right:	Left flow— sit at left:
⎰LH–r 21	⎰RH–l 21
⎱RH–l 1	⎱LH–r 1
RH–l 4	LH–r 4
RH–l 5	LH–r 5
RH–l 6	LH–r 6
RH–r 8	LH–l 8
RH–r 10	LH–l 10
⎰LH–r 19	⎰RH–l 19
⎱RH–r 11	⎱LH–l 11
RH–r 13	LH–l 13
RH–r 14	LH–l 14
LH–r 20	RH–l 20
LH–r 22	RH–l 22
⎰LH–r 23	⎰RH–l 23
⎱RH–r 24	⎱LH–l 24
RH–r 26	LH–l 26
RH–r 27	LH–l 27

Points Used in Regulator Release

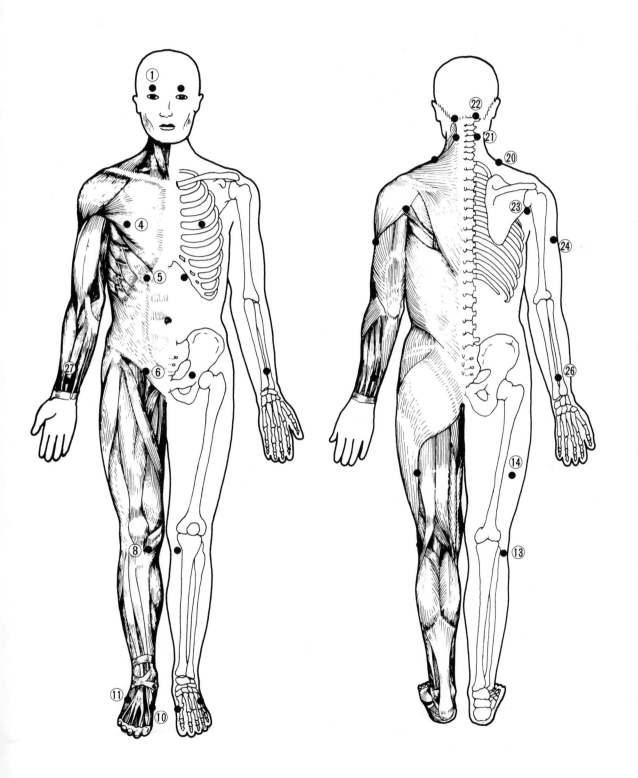

Great Bridge Channel

This treatment pattern is designed to release and balance the Great Bridge Channel in general (see pages 58–59). It helps to balance the body's general energy condition, and was traditionally used for insomnia (concentrating for a longer time on the points of the yang, or posterior, part of the channel) and for drowsiness (concentrating on the yin, or anterior, part of the channel).

This does not mean that a drowsy person will necessarily wake up and be full of energy right after a Jin Shin Do treatment. Especially if a person has spent a lot of time being "all keyed up," balancing his or her energy flows may initiate a desire to sleep as the body asserts its right to a balance between relaxation and work, and to time in which to nourish itself. If the recipient has time to rest or sleep for a while after the treatment, this will be time well spent, for it will allow the renewed and balanced energy flow to work in the body. However, the general effect of a Jin Shin Do treatment is complete, deep relaxation during the treatment and renewed energy afterwards.

The following pattern also helps release the back. It is a good release for the neck and scapula regions, as its base points are ♯ 22 and 23.

Bridge Release:

Right flow— sit at right:	Left flow— sit at left:
{ LH–r 22	{ RH–l 22
{ RH–l 2	{ LH–r 2
RH–l 3	LH–r 3
RH–l 4	LH–r 4
RH–l outside top of pubic bone	LH–r outside top of pubic bone
RH–r 9	LH–l 9
{ LH–r 16	{ RH–l 16
{ RH–r little toe[1]	{ LH–l little toe[1]
RH–r 12	LH–l 12
RH–r 15	LH–l 15
{ LH–r 23	{ RH–l 23
{ RH–r 17	{ LH–l 17
RH–r 18	LH–l 18
RH–r middle finger[1]	LH–l middle finger[1]
RH–r 2	LH–l 2

[1]When the toes or fingers are indicated on treatment patterns, the simplest way of holding them is to just wrap your finger around the entire finger or toe. You may instead holding the finger or toe at the base (above the knuckles) or at the tip.

Points Used in Bridge Release

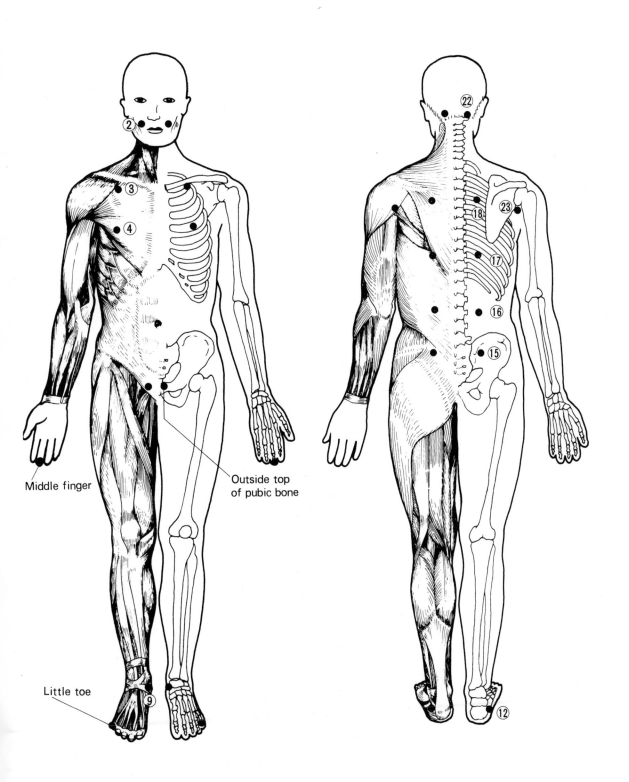

Middle finger

Outside top
of pubic bone

Little toe

Great Central Channel

This treatment pattern is designed to release and balance the Great Central Channel in general (see pages 59–61). The Great Central Channel has perhaps the strongest psychic and spiritual effects of any Strange Flows pair. It is also very important to physical well-being, for the Governing Vessel (yang) flows up the spine while the Conception Vessel (yin) is related to the vital centers of the body.

This treatment pattern may be used as an opening pattern for a treatment session, or it may be used following the release of muscular and energic blocks. As an opener, it helps to relax the person and facilitate spiritual peace and calm.

Central Release:

Sit at the left:

> RH–top of head
> LH–between fifth and sixth thoracic
>   vertebrae
>
> LH–between seventh cervical and
>   first thoracic vertebrae
>
> RH–between seventh cervical and
>   first thoracic vertebrae
> LH–l 9
>
> LH–r 9
>
> LH–l 12
>
> LH–r 12

Sit at the right and continue:

> LH–between first and second lumbar
>   vertebrae
> RH–on top of pubic bone
>
> LH–on sternum (with palm over area)
>
> RH–hara (with palm over area)
>
> LH–hara (with palm over area)
> RH–between second and third lumbar
>   vertebrae
>
> LH–between ninth and tenth thoracic
>   vertebrae
>
> RH–tip of coccyx

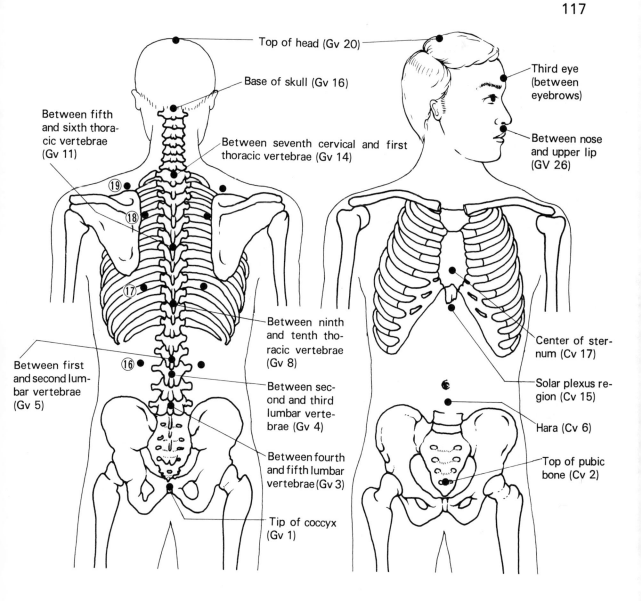

Top of head (Gv 20)

Base of skull (Gv 16)

Between fifth and sixth thoracic vertebrae (Gv 11)

Between seventh cervical and first thoracic vertebrae (Gv 14)

⑲

⑱

⑰

Between first and second lumbar vertebrae (Gv 5)

⑯

Between ninth and tenth thoracic vertebrae (Gv 8)

Between second and third lumbar vertebrae (Gv 4)

Between fourth and fifth lumbar vertebrae (Gv 3)

Tip of coccyx (Gv 1)

Third eye (between eyebrows)

Between nose and upper lip (GV 26)

Center of sternum (Cv 17)

Solar plexus region (Cv 15)

Hara (Cv 6)

Top of pubic bone (Cv 2)

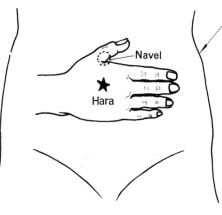

Navel

Hara

Illustration of hand position over the hara in Great Center Release.

The Central Release will be especially powerful if you visualize the flow of ki up the spinal column in the back and down the median line in the front as you do the acupressure release pattern.

Belt and Penetrating Channels

This treatment pattern is designed to
balance and regulate both the Belt and the
Penetrating Channels (see pages 61–62). Because its base points are ♯16 and 6, it is
also a good release for the groin area and
helps release the lower abdomen.

Belt-Penetrating Release:

Right flow—   Left flow—
sit at right: sit at left:

   {LH–r 16   {RH–l 16
   {RH–r 11   {LH–l 11
   RH–r 26   LH–l 26

   {LH–r 6   {RH–l 6
   {RH–r 7   {LH–l 7
   RH–r 8   LH–l 8
   RH–r 10   LH–l 10
   LH–r 27   RH–l 27

Sit at left and   Remain at left and
continue: continue:

   {LH–r top of   {LH–l top of
     pubic bone   pubic bone
   {RH–hara (with {RH–hara (with
     palm over   palm over
     area)   area)
   RH–solar plexus RH–solar plexus
     (palm over   (palm over
     area)   area)
   RH–between   RH–between
     nose and upper   nose and upper
     lip   lip
   RH–third eye   RH–third eye

Both this release and the preceding Central Release are especially effective if the
recipient is directed to practice hara breathing while you do either pattern. However, it
is a good idea to work with hara breathing
meditation yourself for a while before you
show it to others. (See chapter 4.) The releases by themselves are powerful even if
this breathing and meditation technique is
not used.

Points Used in Belt-Penetrating Release

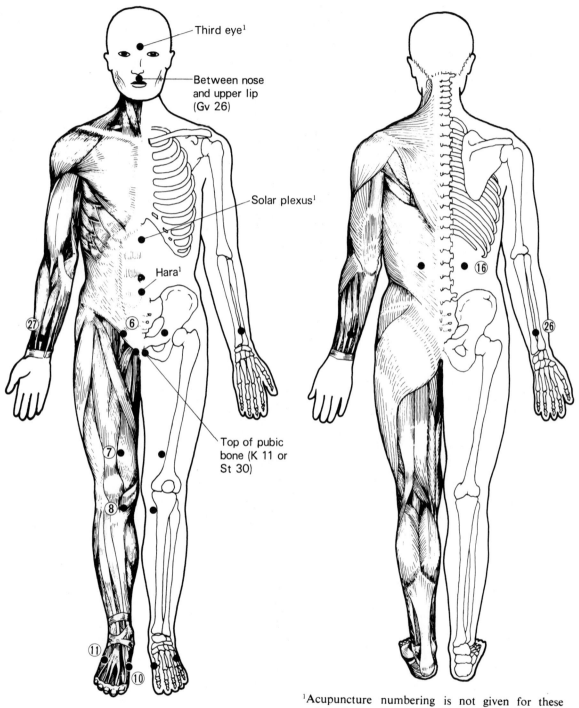

Third eye[1]

Between nose and upper lip (Gv 26)

Solar plexus[1]

Hara[1]

Top of pubic bone (K 11 or St 30)

[1]Acupuncture numbering is not given for these points, because the intent in holding these three points is not to work on acu-points, but rather to direct ki through the palms to the vital centers located internally to the points.

Neck Release

The Jin Shin Do neck release is a thorough bilateral release of the entire neck area—an area which is generally very tense and highly armored, and which, because it is adjacent to the brain, greatly affects our consciousness. If the neck is tense and blocked, the thinking will be less clear, the emotions more cloudy, and the spiritual attitude less free and positive. Because most of the organ meridians and Strange Flow channels pass through this narrow region, it actually influences almost every part of the body. Therefore, releasing this area and directing stagnated ki out of its major points is fundamental.

Releasing the neck at the end of a Jin Shin Do session has a specific purpose, in addition to these general ones. As points on the back and shoulders are released during the acupressure treatment session, some of the ki blocked in these points begins to flow up the Strange Flow channels. If the released ki flowing up the back is impeded by tension at the neck, some of this ki may not be able to continue its journey down the front of the body and to deficient areas. It may stagnate at the already tense neck area, and this increased ki blockage can cause mild dizziness, irritability, or even headache. Simply making a rule of doing a neck release at the end of each session eliminates any possible problems. A good principle to follow during this neck release is that the neck points should be released as much as the back and shoulder points have been.

The following release pattern is a very effective way of working on the neck area; therefore, many students of other massage or release techniques include it in their regular practice as well as in their Jin Shin Do treatments. It may also be used by itself as a short release pattern for this area, when there is not time to do an entire treatment session.

If you are learning Jin Shin Do with your spouse or a friend, exchanging neck release is a marvelous non-verbal communication.

Basic Neck Release:

The basic neck release pattern has already been illustrated (on pages 98–102). In this basic pattern, both hands hold the same point on both sides of the body at the same time. The left hand holds a point on the left side of the body, and the right hand holds the same point on the right side of the body. The hands then move to the succeeding pairs of points at the same time.

Sit at the head:

LH–l 23	and	RH–r 23
LH–l 19	and	RH–r 19
LH–l 20	and	RH–r 20
LH–l 21	and	RH–r 21
LH–l 22	and	RH–r 22

Aids to Neck Release:

To release any of the above points more, or more easily, you may add points from the chart below. Leaving your hand on the tight point that you wish to release further, remove the other hand from the corresponding point on the other side of the body, moving it to hold any appropriate point from the chart. For example, you may be holding both ♯20s. After a couple of minutes, you feel that the right ♯20 has released quite well, but the left ♯20 is still pretty tense. You can leave your left hand on the left ♯20, and move your right hand to hold the left ♯26 and/or the right ♯24. Holding either or both of these points will help the ♯20 to release more quickly and more deeply. Therefore, using points from this chart increases the artistry of the basic neck release.

While holding:	Your other hand may move to:
23	30 (on the same side)
19	26 (on the same side)
20	26 (on the same side) and/or 24 (on the opposite side)
21	5 (on the opposite side)
22	1 (on the opposite or same side)

Points Used in Neck Release

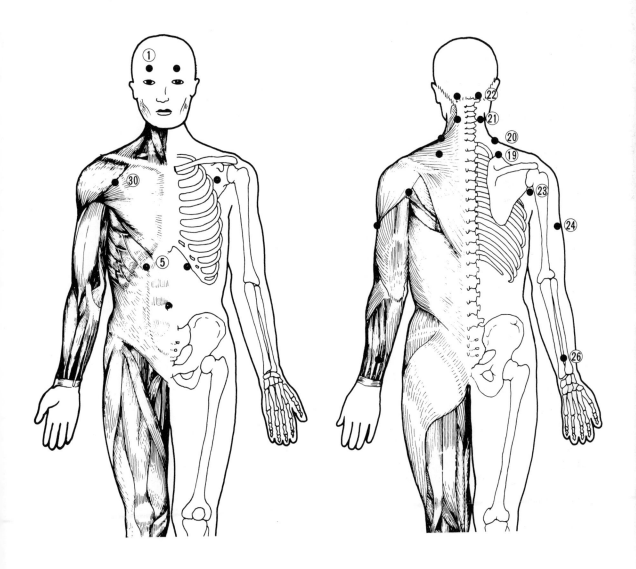

122

End of Treatment Patterns

The end of a treatment is as important as its beginning. Endings in general are as important as beginnings:

> "*What is fragile is easy to break;*
> *What is minute is easy to disperse.*
> *Deal with a thing before it comes into existence;*
> *Regulate a thing before it gets into confusion.*
> *The common people in their business (or affairs and doings) often fail on the verge of succeeding.*
> *Take care with the end as you do with the beginning,*
> *And you will have no failure.*"[1]

At the end of a Jin Shin Do treatment, the person being treated is generally in a very relaxed, peaceful, "high" state. Therefore, the end of the treatment is in many ways the most spiritual part. Your function here is a more subtle regulating of the ki in the vital centers. Your touch should be very light,

your attention concentrated on channeling ki. You may visualize the flow of ki up the back and down the front of the person while you are doing these final steps. Meditate on love and compassion, on a sincere desire for the person's well-being, and on acceptance of whatever is truly necessary for the person being treated.

Centering Release

Do this short pattern after the neck release:

Sit at the head:

{RH–top of head (with fingertips or thumb, or with entire palm)
LH–base of skull
LH–"third eye"
LH–center of sternum between the nipples

---

[1]*Tao Teh Ching*, from Chapter LXIV.

Points Used in Centering Release

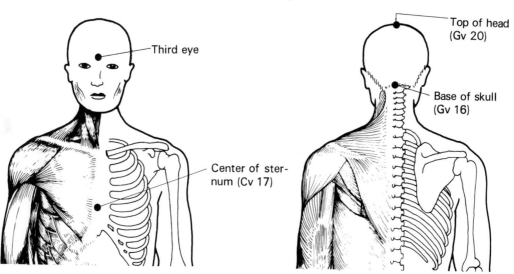

Third eye

Center of sternum (Cv 17)

Top of head (Gv 20)

Base of skull (Gv 16)

Final Balancing Step

Use one of these patterns after the centering release:

Stand or sit at the left:

- RH–center of sternum between nipples (palm over area)
- LH–hara (palm over area)

Stand or sit at the left:

- RH–base of sternum
- LH–both big toes

(See illustration on pages 102–103.)

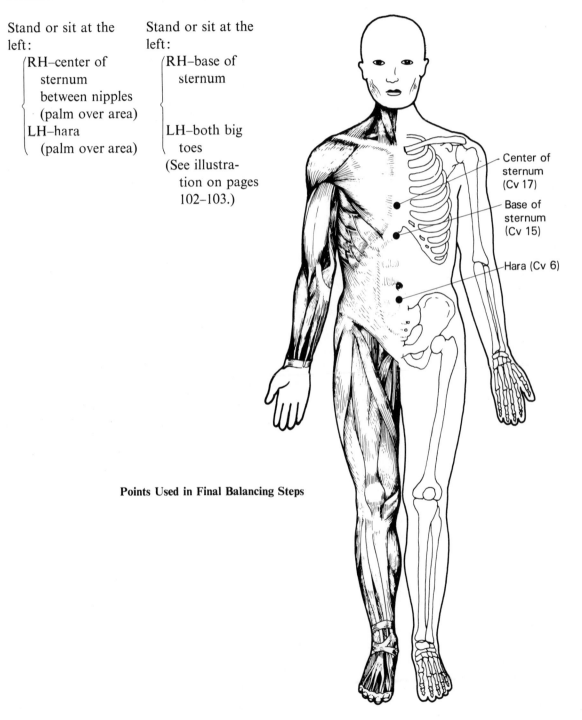

Center of sternum (Cv 17)

Base of sternum (Cv 15)

Hara (Cv 6)

Points Used in Final Balancing Steps

Body Area Release

The following release patterns concentrate on various areas and functions of the body. Yet they are also designed to be general body-mind releases, for in the oriental tradition specifics can only be approached in the context of the whole. These release patterns may be used by themselves or in combination with one or more of the four Strange Flow releases.

Some of these body area releases include one or two new points. These points are all very important general tonic points which are almost universally helpful. The location and the most important traditional associations of each are described as they are introduced.

Basic Back Release

Almost everyone has some chronic tension in one or more of the major flow points along the back. The following release pattern is a good general release for the entire back—points #15 through 19. If any of these points remains especially tight after this release, you may use some other body area release pattern for that particular point, either during the same treatment session or the next time you work on the person.

Right flow— sit at right:	Left flow— sit at left:

{ LH–r 15
{ RH–r behind
  knee
	{ RH–l 15
	{ LH–l behind
	  knee

RH–r 12	LH–l 12
RH–r little toe	LH–l little toe
RH–r 6	LH–l 6
{ LH–r 21 { RH–r 16	{ RH–l 21 { LH–l 16
RH–r 17	LH–l 17
RH–r 18	LH–l 18
LH–r 27	RH–l 27
{ LH–r 19 { RH–r 26	{ RH–l 19 { LH–l 26

{ LH–r 21
{ RH–r tensest
  back point:
  #15, 16, 17,
  or 18
	{ RH–l 21
	{ LH–l tensest
	  back point:
	  #15, 16, 17,
	  or 18

Points Used in Basic Back Release

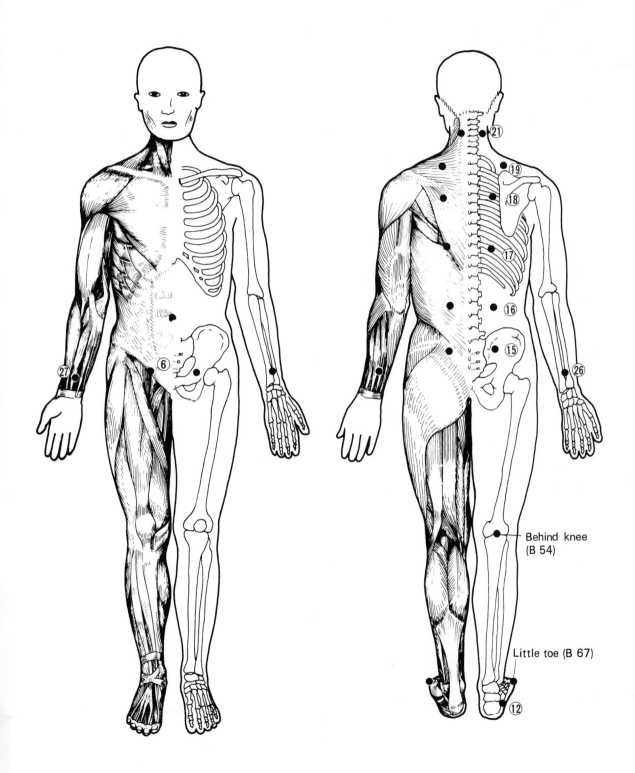

Behind knee (B 54)

Little toe (B 67)

Shoulder Release

This treatment pattern is designed to work on tension throughout the shoulders. It concentrates first on release of #19, and then also of #20 and 30. The #19 is associated with nervous tension and also influences the resistance, the #20 is associated with pressure and frustration, and the #30 with emotional holding. Thus this pattern is a good general body-mind release; it may also be used to help release tension in the arms.

Right flow— sit at right:	Left flow— sit at left:
⌠LH–r 19 ⌡RH–r 23	⌠RH–l 19 ⌡LH–l 23
RH–r 24	LH–l 24
RH–r 25	LH–l 25

RH–r middle,
    ring, and little
    fingers
	LH–l middle,
	    ring, and little
	    fingers

RH–r 16	LH–l 16
LH–r 21	RH–l 21
LH–r 22	RH–l 22
LH–r 20	RH–l 20
RH–r 26	LH–l 26
RH–l 24	LH–r 24
LH–r 30	RH–l 30

RH–r index
    finger and
    thumb
	LH–l index
	    finger and
	    thumb

Points Used in Shoulder Release

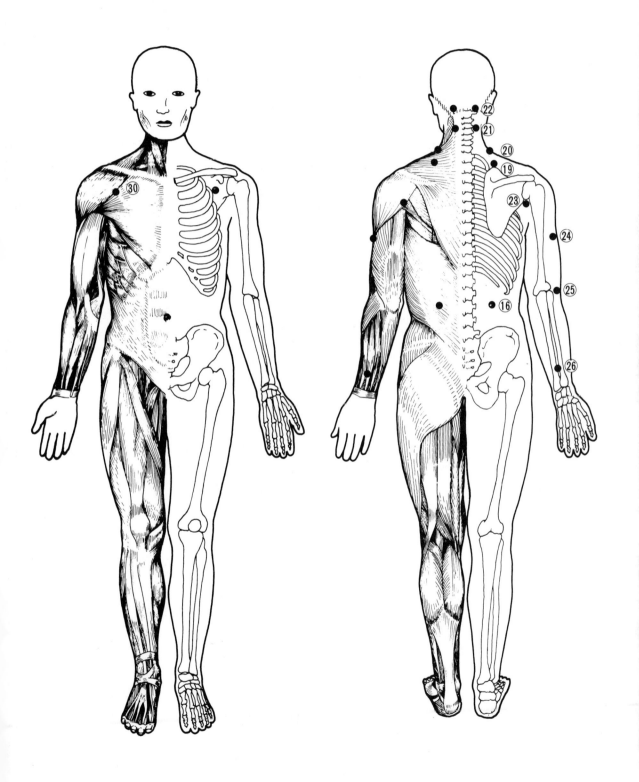

Clear Thinking Release

This is a good pattern to use if the person being treated has the most tension in the neck—around ♯22, 21, or 20—or has a headache. In the latter case, do the pattern for the tensest side first, as usual. Then, holding each point for a shorter time, it may be helpful to also do the other side. If you do both the right and left versions of this release pattern, you need not follow it with the neck release unless you wish to work on the area more. Instead, just finish with the end of treatment steps.

Right flow— sit at right:	Left flow— sit at left:
{LH–r 22	{RH–l 22
{RH–l 11	{LH–r 11
RH–l 13	LH–r 13
RH–l 14	LH–r 14
{LH–r 21	{RH–l 21
{RH–l 9	{LH–r 9
RH–l 12	LH–r 12
{LH–r 19	{RH–l 19
{RH–r 24	{LH–l 24
LH–r 20	RH–l 20
RH–r 26	LH–l 26
RH–l 1	LH–r 1
LH–r 22	RH–l 22

The Clear Thinking Release may be followed with this additional step, visualizing the ki flow up the cervical (neck) vertebrae, over the head, and down the front of the body along the Great Central Channel.

Sit at the left:

{ LH–between first thoracic and seventh cervical vertebrae
{ RH–base of skull (above first cervical vertebra)

Points Used in Clear Thinking Release

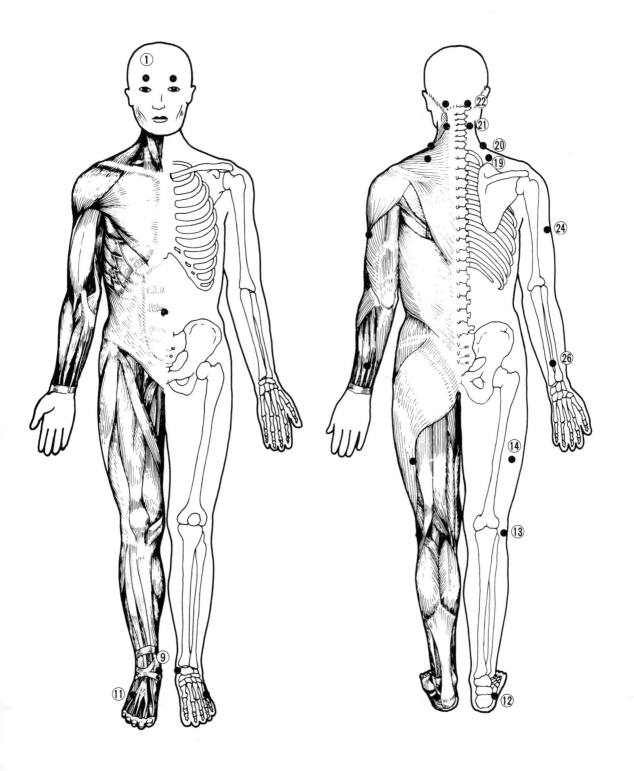

Points Used in Abdominal Release

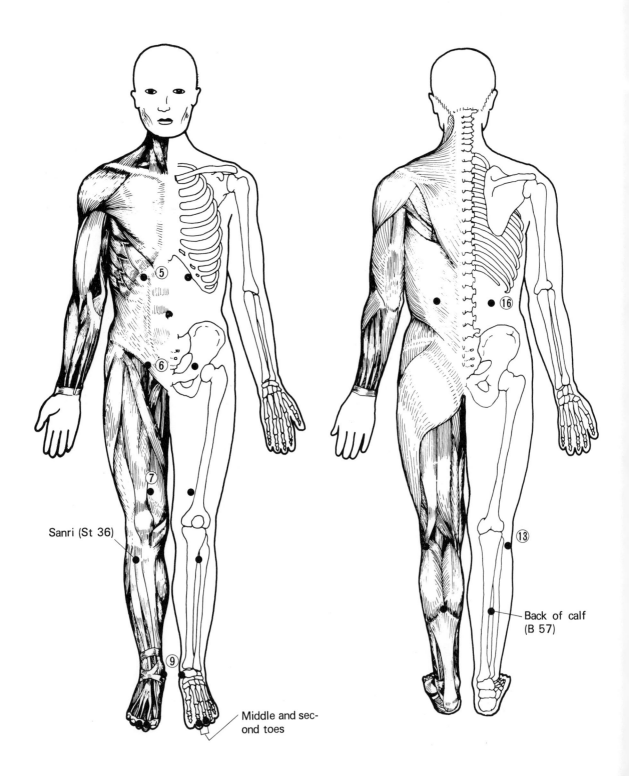

Sanri (St 36)

Middle and second toes

Back of calf (B 57)

Abdominal Release

The following treatment pattern is based on points traditionally used to help release abodominal discomfort, indigestion, and constipation. It is therefore helpful for common flu, upset stomach, and intestinal gas, and is a good general release for the abdominal area.

Right flow— sit at right:

{ LH–r 16
{ RH–r 5
RH–r 6
RH–l 7
RH–r 9
RH–r 13

Left flow— sit at left:

{ RH–l 16
{ LH–l 5
LH–l 6
LH–r 7
LH–l 9
LH–l 13

Follow this with these additional steps, preferably doing both the right and the left versions of each. These may also be used by themselves as short, quick release patterns for the abdominal area.

Right flow— sit at the feet:

{ LH–r 12
{ RH–r back of
{   calf

{ RH–r middle
{   and second
{   toes together
{   (hold at base
{   of toes)
{ LH–r sanri

Left flow— sit at the feet:

{ RH–l 12
{ LH–l back of
{   calf

{ LH–l middle
{   and second
{   toes together
{   (hold at base
{   of toes)
{ RH–l sanri

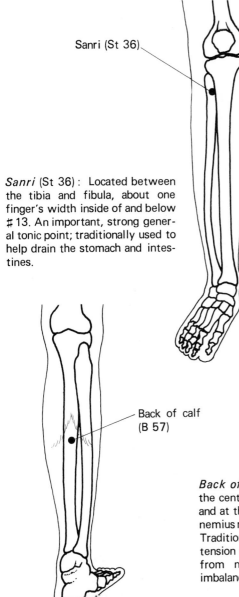

Sanri (St 36)

Sanri (St 36) : Located between the tibia and fibula, about one finger's width inside of and below ♯ 13. An important, strong general tonic point; traditionally used to help drain the stomach and intestines.

Back of calf (B 57)

Back of Calf (B 57) : Located in the center of the back of the calf, and at the bottom of the gastrocnemius muscle (fleshy part of calf). Traditionally used for abdominal tension and queasiness, especially from nervousness or emotional imbalance.

Points Used in Deep Breathing Release

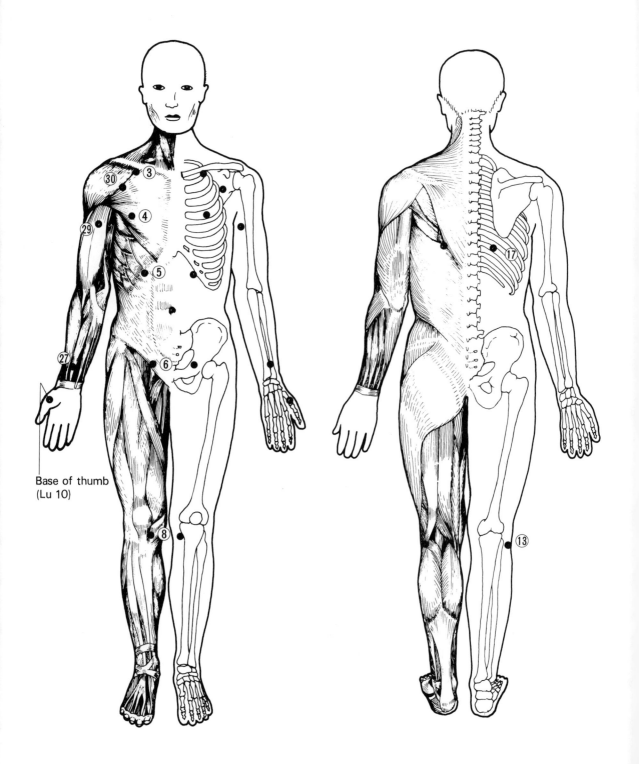

Base of thumb
(Lu 10)

Deep Breathing Release

The following pattern is designed to facilitate free and complete respiration—both abdominal and chest breathing. Before you begin this release pattern, notice how the person is breathing. Many people will be breathing only through the chest; the abdomen will remain rigid and unmoving because the diaphragm is tense. The first three lines of the pattern especially help to release diaphragm tension. To release the diaphragm further, you may guide the person to do basic hara breathing while you do this release.

If the diaphragm is moving freely in respiration, the internal organs will be forced downward by its movement and the abdomen will expand visibly during the inhalation. Hara breathing meditation is still good as almost everyone needs to center more completely in the hara and to fill it with ki. The exhalation may be through the nose rather than through the mouth, when hara breathing is practiced within a treatment session.

Right flow— sit at right:	Left flow— sit at left:
⌠LH–r 17	⌠RH–l 17
⌡RH–r 5	⌡LH–l 5
RH–l 13	LH–r 13
⌠LH–r 18	⌠RH–l 18
⌡RH–r 3	⌡LH–l 3
RH–r 6	LH–l 6
RH–l 8	LH–r 8
RH–r 27	LH–l 27
RH–r 29	LH–l 29
LH–r 30	RH–l 30
RH–r base of thumb	LH–l base of thumb
RH–r 4	LH–l 4

Base of thumb (Lu 10)

Base of Thumb (Lu 10): Located behind the head of the first metacarpal and in the fleshy part of the base of the thumb, at the tender point. An important point of the lung meridian, traditionally used to facilitate free breathing.

134

Variations on the Deep Breathing Release

1. If the nose is blocked, you may do the following short pattern instead of or before the first three lines of Deep Breathing Release at preceding page.

Right flow—   Left flow—
sit at right: sit at left:

{RH–r 2   {LH–l 2
{LH–r 21   {RH–l 21
 LH–r 22   RH–l 22

This should, of course, be supplemented by other means of taking care of a cold naturally, including extra rest, adequate nourishment, enough liquids, and abstinence from tense situations!

2. The following short pattern may be used to help increase the resistance to external "evils," including the effects of climatic change and of climatic extremes such as cold and wind. It is based on points traditionally used to help reduce fever and hasten recovery from colds. It may be used instead of or before the first three lines of Deep Breathing Release at preceding page.

Right flow—   Left flow—
sit at right: sit at left:

{LH–r 19   {RH–l 19
{RH–r 25   {LH–l 25
 RH–r hoku   LH–l hoku
 RH–r each   LH–l each
   fingertip   fingertip

Points Used in Variations

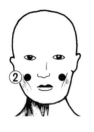

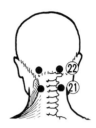

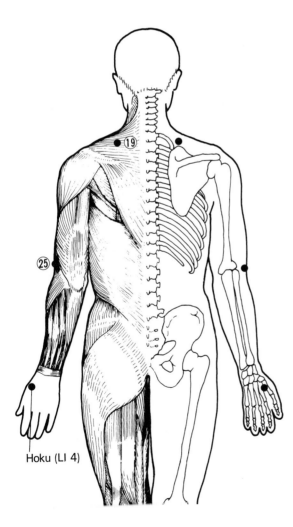

Hoku (LI 4)

Hoku (LI 4): Located on the outside of the hand between the thumb and index fingers. just below the junction of the first and second metacarpals. It is an important general tonic point, and was traditionally used for constipation, fever, and colds. It should not be used on pregnant women.

Hoku (LI 4)

Potency Treatment

This release pattern is particularly good for men, but is also an excellent release for the lower back area, especially the region of #16.

Right flow—
sit at right:

{LH–r 16
{RH–l 13
RH–l 12
RH–l 11
RH–l each toe,
    from little
    to big
{RH–r 16
{LH–r 23
RH–r 11

Left flow—
sit at left:

{RH–l 16
{LH–r 13
LH–r 12
LH–r 11
LH–r each toe,
    from little
    to big
{LH–l 16
{RH–l 23
LH–l 11

As a release pattern to promote the natural functioning of the male sexual system, the above pattern may be preceded with or followed by this short pattern:

Right flow—
sit at right:

{LH–r 15
{RH–l 8
RH–l 9
LH–r 18

Left flow—
sit at left:

{RH–l 15
{LH–r 8
LH–r 9
RH–l 18

Sit at the right
and continue:

{RH–r side of
{ sacrum
{LH–above
{ pubic bone
{LH–between
{ second and
{ third lumbar
{ vertebrae
{RH–between
{ fourth and
{ fifth·lumbar
{ vertebrae

Sit at the right
and continue:

{RH–l side of
{ sacrum
{LH–above
{ pubic bone
{LH–between
{ second and
{ third lumbar
{ vertebrae
{RH–between
{ fourth and
{ fifth lumbar
{ vertebrae

Points Used in Potency Treatment

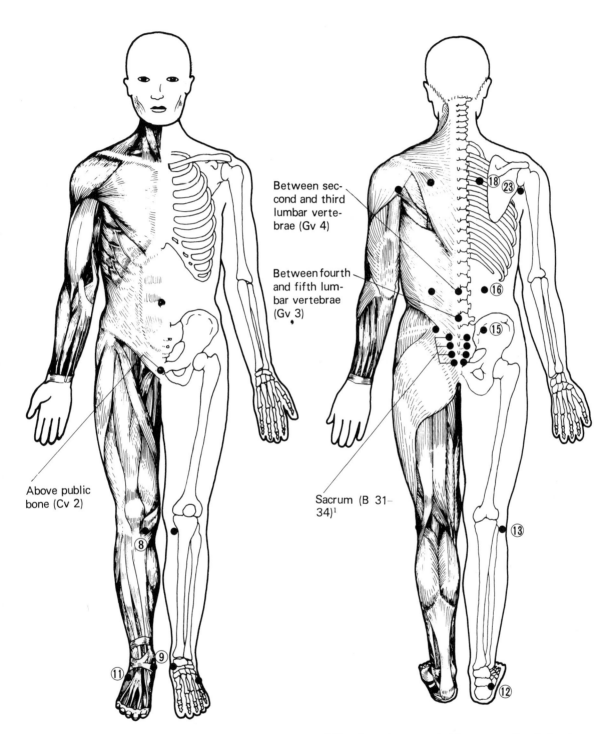

Between seccond and third lumbar vertebrae (Gv 4)

Between fourth and fifth lumbar vertebrae (Gv 3)

Above public bone (Cv 2)

Sacrum (B 31–34)[1]

[1]The fingertips may hold any or all of the four points shown on the sacrum.

Points Used in Female Regulating Release

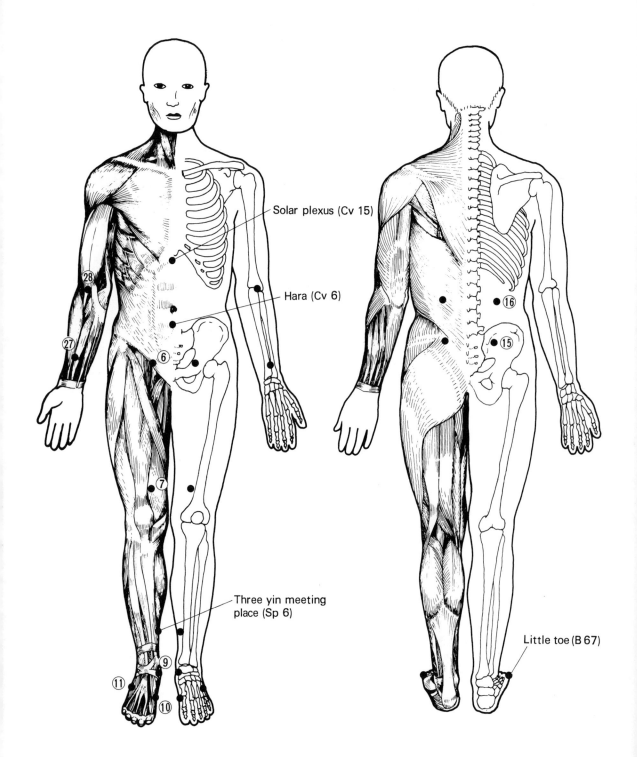

Solar plexus (Cv 15)

Hara (Cv 6)

Three yin meeting place (Sp 6)

Little toe (B 67)

Female Regulating Release

The natural functioning of the female system is fundamental to a woman's health. Therefore, this pattern should not be regarded as just a symptomatic treatment for the female organs, but rather as a balancing and releasing treatment for her vital functioning as a woman. To experience this life completely, the balancing of both the general physical and energic condition, as well as the physical and energic capabilities particular to each sex, is necessary. The latter generally takes place after the rest of the system is fairly healthy, for Nature is concerned with nourishing the individual before providing for procreation.

Right flow—sit at right:	Left flow—sit at left:
{ LH–r 16	{ RH–l 16
{ RH–r 9	{ LH–l 9
RH–r little toe	LH–l little toe
{ LH–r 6	{ RH–l 6
{ RH–l 7	{ LH–r 7
RH–l three yin meeting place	LH–r three yin meeting place
{ LH–r 15	{ RH–l 15
{ RH–l 10	{ LH–r 10
RH–l 11	LH–r 11
RH–r 7	LH–l 7
LH–r 27	RH–l 27
LH–r 28	RH–l 28

Sit at the left and continue:	Sit at the left and continue:
{ RH–solar plexus (palm over area)	{ RH–solar plexus (palm over area)
{ LH–hara (palm over area)	{ LH–hara (palm over area)

Three Yin Meeting Place (Sp 6): Located just behind the tibia and about four fingers' width above the inner anklebone (malleolus). Traditionally used for the female organs and to strengthen the general condition of women and men. This point should not be used on pregnant women.

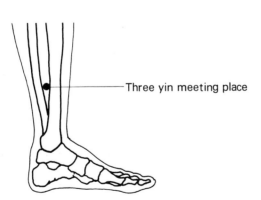
Three yin meeting place

General Yin Sei Release

This is a good treatment pattern to use for someone whose overall condition (sei) is basically too yin. You may follow this release with some particular body area release; however, just doing the following pattern plus the neck release and ending steps would be a good treatment format. Refer to the section "The Yin and Yang of our Physical Conditions" in chapter 3 for a description of the yin condition, and for suggestions as to acupressure technique.

Sit at the left:

<blockquote>

RH–top of head
LH–between second and third lumbar vertebrae
LH–between ninth and tenth thoracic vertebrae
LH–between seventh cervical and first thoracic vertebrae
RH–below protrusion at back of skull

</blockquote>

Right flow— sit at right:	Left flow— sit at left:
LH–r 18	RH–l 18
RH–r 27	LH–l 27
LH–r 3	RH–l 3
RH–r sanri	LH–l sanri
LH–r 21	RH–l 21
RH–l 1	LH–r 1
LH–r 22	RH–l 22
RH–top of sternum	LH–top of sternum
LH–r side of pubic bone	RH–l side of pubic bone
RH–r 9	LH–l 9
LH–r 16	LH–l 16
RH–l 5	LH–r 5
LH–r 6	RH–l 6
RH–r 8	LH–l 8
RH–r 10	LH–l 10

141

Points Used in General Yin Sei Release

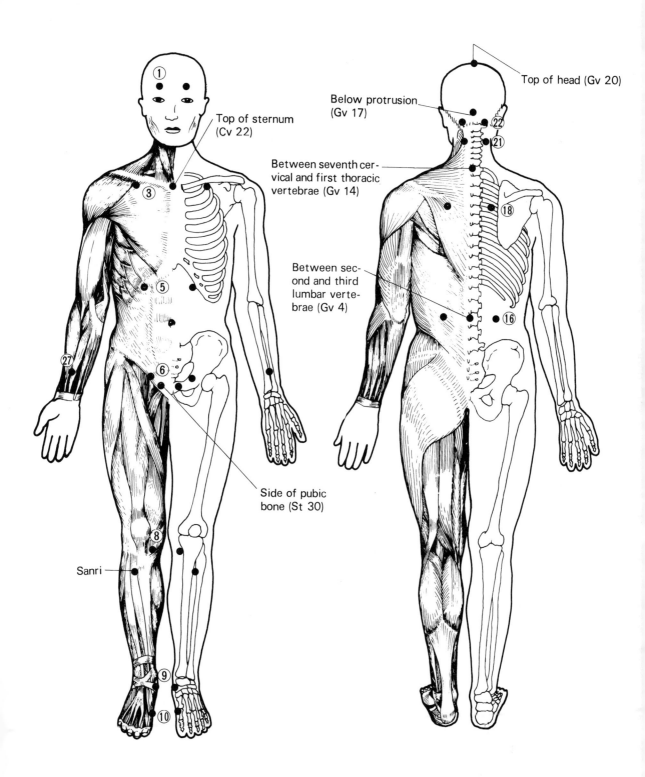

Top of sternum (Cv 22)

Below protrusion (Gv 17)

Top of head (Gv 20)

Between seventh cervical and first thoracic vertebrae (Gv 14)

Between second and third lumbar vertebrae (Gv 4)

Side of pubic bone (St 30)

Sanri

142

General Yang Sei Release

This is a good treatment pattern to use for someone whose overall condition (sei) is basically too yang. Since this is a fairly long pattern, just doing, it plus the neck release and ending steps, is a good treatment format. Refer to the section "The Yin and Yang of our Physical Condition" in chapter 3, for a description of the yang condition and for suggestions as to acupressre technique.

Sit at the left:

   {RH–top of head
   {LH–tip of coccyx
   LH–between fourth and fifth lumbar vertebrae
   LH–between seventh and eighth thoracic vertebrae.
   LH–base of skull
   LH–center of sternum

Right flow—sit at right:	Left flow—sit at left:
{LH–r 23 {RH–l 11	{RH–l 23 {LH–r 11
RH–r 24	LH–l 24
LH–r 20	RH–l 20
RH–r 13	LH–l 13
LH–r 19	RH–l 19
RH–r 26	LH–l 26
RH–r each fingertip	LH–l each fingertip
{LH–r 15 {RH–r 12	{RH–l 15 {LH–l 12
LH–r 16	RH–l 16
RH–r each toe at tip	LH–l each toe at tip
RH–r behind knee	LH–l behind knee
LH–r 17	RH–l 17
LH–r 18	RH–l 18
{LH–r 21 and 22 {RH–l 1	{RH–l 21 and 22 {LH–r 1
RH–top of the sternum	LH–top of sternum
RH–l 4	LH–r 4

Points Used in General Yang Sei Release

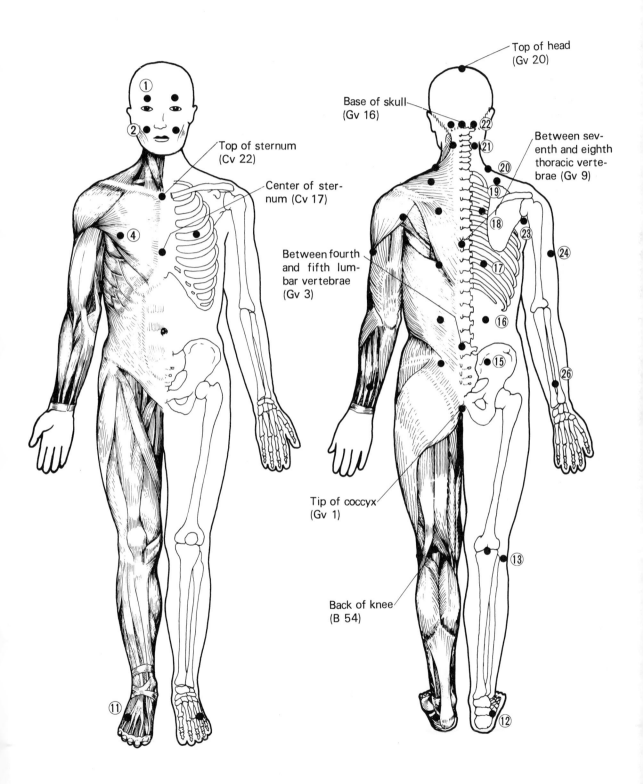

Top of head
(Gv 20)

Base of skull
(Gv 16)

Top of sternum
(Cv 22)

Center of ster-
num (Cv 17)

Between sev-
enth and eighth
thoracic verte-
brae (Gv 9)

Between fourth
and fifth lum-
bar vertebrae
(Gv 3)

Tip of coccyx
(Gv 1)

Back of knee
(B 54)

9. AN ANCIENT, NEW AGE APPROACH TO THE EMOTIONS

One of the most primary alienations is the body/mind separation—the tendency to regard body and mind as two separate entities. For example, we say: "My back is bothering me," "This arm is giving me trouble," If I could just get rid of my shoulder tension," "If this headache would just leave me alone." And so we look for the perfect panacea that will instantly and magically dissolve our aches and pains, our weaknesses and fatigues. But there simply is no perfect panacea. Both physical and emotional causes of our problems must be considered, and we must learn to take physical and emotional responsibility for our own conditions.

This is the real magic. Not just symptomatic relief, wonderful as that may be. Not just release, if we are still thinking "I am releasing my body tensions." Not even just awareness, in the sense of "I" being aware of "my" mental processes, emotional makeup, physical condition, or even spiritual being. The real magic is discovering and experiencing the whole inter-twined spiral of body and mind, feelings and emotions, thoughts and intuitions or revelations. All of it. All of me. We must move out of our heads—out of our analytical and limited conceptions of self—and into our entire being.

Where are the boundaries of the "self"? As we become aware of our tensions and blocks, experience the wonderful feeling of releasing these, feel the flow of ki through our bodies, and get in touch with our vital centers, we begin to experience our being in every cell of our body. Our conception of the self changes. As we give Jin Shin Do treatments and experience the infinite plasticity or change-ability of the energy body, and of the entire body-mind, our conception of the self continues to shift radically. We begin to feel the unity of body and mind and, further, the energy connections that exist between ourselves and other beings—and indeed between all living beings in the great universal ocean of ki. We discover that besides being internally one, "I" am also not separate from others or from my environment.

Homo sapiens is almost like those science fiction races in which all the "individuals" are not separate but are really cells of one larger being, cells which constantly communicate with and influence each other and thus the whole. We experience this unity constantly—or rather, being unconscious of its effects, we allow it to influence us constantly.

In personal interactions, people of weak energy can unconsciously or consciously drain or sap the energy of those with whom they communicate. Persons of strong energy, on the other hand, can raise or lower the energy of an entire area—a group of friends, a family, business, school, or neighborhood—depending on their clarity or cloudiness. Sensitive persons can tune into and be strongly influenced by the emotional and energic conditions of other persons, even in such casual encounters as supermarket shopping or party-going. Unless these individuals are in touch with their own centers, they can even begin to experience the emotional and spiritual states of those they come in contact with. Anxiety, paranoia, fear, suspicion, worry—these and other imbalanced emotional states are contagious. But we can control the contagion by exploring ourselves and developing a strong sense of our own inner natures.

Alternatives to Armoring

Body "armoring" is deep physical tension which tends to re-create or create associated emotional imbalance. To armor or tense is to resist. But in resisting, we try to avoid a feeling or emotion we are already experiencing! We are already feeling anger, fear, or even love before we begin trying to repress those feelings. We are likewise already experiencing physical pain, soreness, or strain before we begin trying to avoid those sensations. The essence of armoring is an attempt to numb ourselves, so that we cease to feel the unpleasant. Rather than accepting and exploring our feelings, we resist and try to stop them.

But our feelings and emotions are not mechanical things which can be turned on and off. Neither are they uncontrollable forces which needs must take us hither and thither. We do not always need to translate our feelings into all of the actions that they might imply. But neither need we resist acting on the basis of our feelings as opposed to our minds. Emotions and feelings animate and enrich our lives, as long as they are in general balanced and controlled by Shin— our inner Spirit.

We have two basic alternatives: armoring and openness. Armoring doesn't work. As we try to harden ourselves against experiences, we just incorporate our feelings further into our structures. Associated areas of the body tighten; the physical tension deepens and hardens; and our bodies actually become records of our intellectual, emotional, spiritual, physical, and energic experiences. Pain, grief, fear, anger, worry—all of these are still there, within us. We simply push them down to a sub-conscious level so that we need not continue consciously experiencing them—and so that we need not deal with them.

As a result, the more we armor, the more depressed, irritable, frustrated, worried, and unhappy we become. Life loses its color and flavor, and becomes a monotonous routine. Waking up—in the morning or throughout the day—becomes difficult. We cease to greet each new day with pleasure, joy, and appreciation. Eventually, we either explode, become very depressed, or just go to sleep. We cease to grow, to become ourselves. We stop unfolding or uncovering our inner Spirits and start just reacting to the surrounding social mores, which we have incorporated into our own bodies and minds—often while detesting or hating those very things. Attempting to shut out pain, we instead shut out pleasure and joy.

The other alternative—openness—is more scary at first, for its other name is Freedom. But if we think back to the times we were happiest, the times we tend to reminisce about, these were usually the times when we felt the most free. Not free in the sense of having no responsibilities or obligations, but free in the sense that we were in touch with Shin and its desires—feeling the outflowing of our inner Spirit and the inflowing of the universal spiritual energy.

Can we allow ourselves to choose the alternative of openness? Can we allow ourselves to discover and acknowledge our armorings? This is the same as asking whether or not we really have faith in the Tao, which is the same as asking whether or not we truly appreciate life and all its cycles. If we understand Lao Tzu's three—the spirallic alternation of yin and yang, and the all-pervading ki—not just intellectually but in the very practical and real way of the ancient oriental people, we see that there truly is nothing to be feared but fear itself. What we need comes, and what we do not need is taken away. Sometimes we have to pay our dues, and sometimes we get dessert. The bigger the back, the bigger the front. By armoring, we make this process more difficult and traumatic, but we never can successfully stop it.

The river of life is very much stronger than the rivers of the world. We can, with modern technology or technological pollution, wreak disastrous effects on our earthly rivers, but we cannot stop them from flowing. How, then, can we think that we can stop the river of life? This river—the Big I—is so very much stronger than the ego—the little i. It demands from us awe and reverence. It should automatically call forth from us awe and reverence and appreciation, rather than resistance. But resistance is our heritage.

I had a very funky experience during the writing of this book which, though insignificant in a way, strongly affected me. It occurred after a series of experiences in which what I did not appreciate was simply taken away. I was living in a house on top of a city hill, and the only way of getting up to that house was by climbing 95 steps. 95 steps with groceries, pet food, or a sleeping four-year-old child in your arms is a lot of steps! It made me stronger—but it also often drained my energies. One afternoon I had complained my way up about two-thirds of the steps, feeling generally rebellious and bitchy. Just as I had really worked my resentment up to a climactic pitch, my right foot landed in a large pile of dog excrement. All I could do was laugh and think, "OK already! I finally got the message!" Appre-

ciate, appreciate, appreciate. Everything. Difficulties and desserts.

Simultaneously, the other task at hand is to get rid of our armoring and blocks, to stop working against our greater selves, to get out of the ruts that keep us down, and to start realizing our potential for facilitating our self-becoming and growth. If we continuously open our energy channels, become more and more aware of our physical and emotional conditions, thoughts and feelings can enter our consciousness, be recognized in their reality, acted upon if necessary, and let go of.

Almost everyone has some chronic tension, or armoring, in one or more of the major flow points; in fact, some regions may be so highly armored as to resemble an armadillo! What could we resemble instead, were we to choose the alternative of openness? If you pet or massage an un-neurotic cat or dog, you will notice that its muscular condition is very different from the typical human being's. When the animal is resting, its muscles are soft and flexible. Yet two seconds later it can be running up a hill faster than we can imagine running on a flat stretch. This is the condition we can aspire to: both strength and flexibility, the ability to use our bodies and minds efficiently and to relax both completely.

The longer we are immersed in the problems and pressures of the material world, forgetting the world of the Spirit, the deeper are the layers of armoring that develop. The more we try to repress our feelings and hide our emotions, the more we feel like the victims rather than initiators of change. Rather than riding the waves of change, we are continuously trying to catch up with them. So they sweep over us and knock us down. Deep armoring, with its old emotional content, prevents us from living in the here-and-now, for it incorporates the past into our very being. Although we may wish to respond freely and freshly to each new situation, we cannot do so as long as the old response patterns are locked into our physical structures.

"*The more restrictions and avoidances*
are in the empire,
The poorer become the people;
The more sharp implements the people
keep,
The more confusions are in the country;
The more arts and crafts men have,
The more are fantastic things produced;
The more laws and regulations are given,
The more robbers and thieves there
are..."[1]

"*There is no greater crime than seeking*
what men desire;
There is no greater misery than knowing
no content;
There is no greater calamity than in-
dulging in greed.
Therefore the contentment of knowing
content will ever be contented."[2]

The Emotions and Ki

According to the ancient oriental teachers, the kaleidoscopic shifting of the emotions is a natural response to the changes of our environment—to both people and events, places and problems. But often we stop this natural response process by holding onto an emotion—trying to stop the river of change. The repressed emotion is automatically imbalanced, for it is stagnant. This imbalanced emotion—worry, fear, grief, anger, or some other favorite—begins to control our whole being. Arising from the conflict between our inner desires and the demands we feel from our social environment, the imbalanced emotion replaces Shin as the ruler of body and mind. Eventually, its control affects all parts of the self.

There is one very simple way to help balance our emotional condition. It can be used at any time and place, and during the experience of almost any emotional distress —especially when that distress is related to the actions or attitudes (real or imagined) of others. Since our emotional responses may in fact be appropriate, it is all right to express what we are feeling! Preferably, of course, with the intention of helping rather than hurting another person. Expressing does not mean expelling all over someone else, unless that person is your therapist or someone who has agreed to be a lay therapist to you.

Women have generally been trained not to express anger, a yang emotion (or even its balanced manifestation, assertiveness). Men have often been trained not to express sorrow, fear, or other yin emotions. But we can learn to say: "I feel angry that ...," "I fear that ...," "I feel hurt that ...," etc. Also, as an antidote, "I love you"—and not just to our mates but also, at least by gestures and actions, to friends, relatives, and associates. As we listen to our inner Spirits (rather than to the universal worries) and express our feelings, we allow ourselves a safety valve. Explosions or depressions—the most extreme and debilitating imbalances —occur more rarely and with less intensity. Also, armoring is dissolved almost before it develops, and often deeper levels of communication are reached.

What happens to our ki when our emotional conditions become imbalanced? The oriental sages described seven primary imbalanced emotions which affect the ki in different ways. It is important to note that these effects occur even if we repress the emotion. So the ki imbalances described below can be acute or chronic.

---

[1] *Tao Teh Ching*, from Chapter LVII.
[2] *Ibid.*, from Chapter XLVI.

1. Anger

In anger the ki "rushes up," concentrating in the shoulders, neck, and upper arms. There may be so much energy blocked here that we feel like pressure cookers and cannot think clearly. Sometimes, the stimulation that anger gives to our physical systems—the unleashing of adrenalin and the resultant desire to act—is necessary and helpful. But often, especially within civilization, excessive anger only makes it more difficult for us to see situations clearly and to solve our problems.

We can use a simple breathing exercise to help release and expel anger, so that the energy unleashed by anger can be directed into appropriate channels and made available for our use. First inhale slowly and deeply, into the hara, imagining that with the breath you are also inhaling all your angers, frustrations, and irritations. Then exhale rapidly through your mouth, loudly saying "BAH!" at the same time, and visualizing the internalized feelings and pressures leaving with the "BAH!" exhalation.

Some classic techniques for getting rid of anger are hitting a pillow (and visualizing it as the person or situation that angers you), or having a pillow fight (not necessarily with the person you are angry with). Physical work is another good way to channel the anger energy in order to clear the mind and center the emotions. Working off anger through running, cleaning the house, playing tennis or volleyball, hitting a tether ball, or performing any other vigorous physical activity allows the body to make use of the rush of adrenalin and helps direct the ki out of the shoulder-neck area.

Chronic tension in these areas suggests that we may have held in the emotion of anger. The resultant frozen, tense musculature cannot only be released by reflection. The body and mind are one: besides acknowledging and doing something about the situation that angers us, we must also release and use the blocked energy. Otherwise, when anger is bottled up inside of us, it becomes self-destructive.

Acu-points for Anger[1]

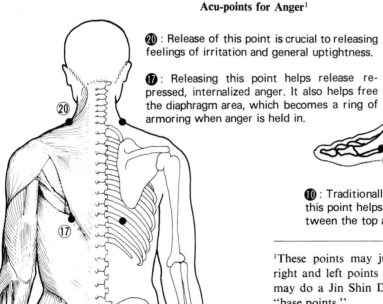

20: Release of this point is crucial to releasing feelings of irritation and general uptightness.

17: Releasing this point helps release repressed, internalized anger. It also helps free the diaphragm area, which becomes a ring of armoring when anger is held in.

10: Traditionally used for anger and rage, this point helps eliminate gaps of ki between the top and bottom of the body.

[1]These points may just be held bilaterally (both right and left points at the same time) or else you may do a Jin Shin Do Release in which these are "base points."

2. Grief

Grief can be a necessary and helpful experience, for essentially grief is letting go of something or someone that is lost to us. If loss is understood and accepted, perhaps grief will not be so intense or unbearable. But when experiences are stronger than our individual wills or understandings, we must often let go on a physical as well as a cerebral level. Crying is the natural physical release. Another person's sympathy, a hand to hold, may be all that is necessary to enable us to let go in this way.

In very traumatic or distressing situations, sometimes our grief is so strong that we cannot let go enough or quickly enough, and we hold onto or repress some of our feelings. Grief may "well up inside us," but we cannot release it all—and may not even be conscious of it. At such times, acupressure release such as that described below can turn night to day in terms of emotional well-being.

Basically, in grief the ki is dispersed and the body is weakened. After grieving, we must nourish ourselves and rebuild our ki. Any or all of the Jin Shin Do practices can help us on the way to renewed vitality.

Acu-points for Grief

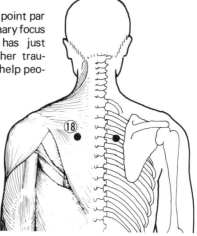

30 : This is the "letting go" point par excellence. It should be a primary focus of release when a person has just experienced loss or some other trauma, and can also be used to help people let go in general.

18 : This point helps to strengthen the body after the experience of grief.

3. Fear

In fear, the ki is drained, descending to the bowels and lower extremities. Often the legs feel weak or shaky, and in extreme fear there may even be urinary incontinence. The feeling is of the energy, or ki, leaking out.

One of the best remedial exercises for fear is hara breathing. This will fill the hara and vital centers with ki and center the body ki, helping to transmute fear into resolution. Hara breathing also initiates relaxed responses to situations and allows us to regain control of ourselves.

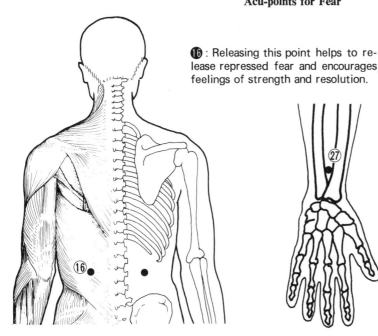

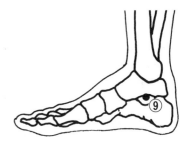

16 : Releasing this point helps to release repressed fear and encourages feelings of strength and resolution.

9 : This point can be used for stage fright or fears about any kind of performance.

27 : This point was traditionally used for fear, especially if one is frightened easily.

4. Worry

Worry "coagulates the ki," in effect paralyzing the body or the ability to act. When we are worried, we usually find it difficult to get much done. We cannot work as effectively. Projects go more slowly. We trip over our own minds—and may in fact be accident-prone. When we feel free and are not worried, often we amaze ourselves with the amount that we have accomplished in a single day, or the many things we have cleared up.

Acu-points for Worry

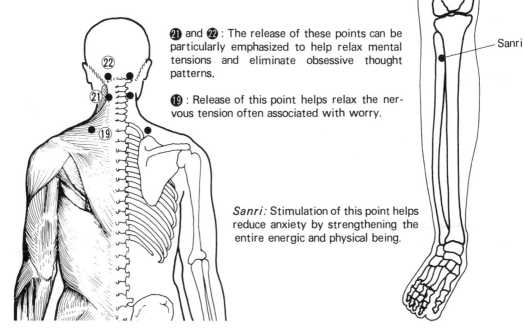

Any Jin Shin Do acupressure release patterns help to release, move, and generally un-coagulate the ki !

21 and **22** : The release of these points can be particularly emphasized to help relax mental tensions and eliminate obsessive thought patterns.

19 : Release of this point helps relax the nervous tension often associated with worry.

Sanri: Stimulation of this point helps reduce anxiety by strengthening the entire energic and physical being.

Sanri

There are a couple main types of worry. One type is mental stress and overthinking. Our minds get hold of something and worry it like a terrier dog teasing a bone. Another type is a feeling of pervasive uneasiness and anxiety, and is often the result of draining emotional stress and physical fatigue.

An antidote to the over-thinking variety of worry is non-thinking—meditating, playing or listening to music, making or appreciating arts or crafts, dancing or exercising. Anything that gets us out of our heads and into other parts of our being. Just getting away from the environment or persons associated with the worry can help change the emotional pattern, so that the mind can see the forest (the overall picture) instead of just the trees (all its aspects and ramifications).

Antidotes to the second variety, anxiety, include just extra rest, nourishing food, and health practices for building the general body ki. Hara breathing is helpful both for relieving acute attacks of anxiety, and also for transmuting a chronic anxious state back to a balanced emotional state of being—which includes a feeling of inner strength and also a sense of humor! When the energy is strong, the person feels more clear, and it is much easier to let go of worries.

5. Reminiscence

Reminiscence concentrates the ki in the brain. In dreaming of or wishing for the past, we are in effect living within our heads, where the past is being experienced. Though it can be pleasurable, reminiscence can become chronic. Especially in reminiscing about the path not taken, the relationship not begun or continued, or the times gone by, we can become so preoccupied with the past that we cease to fully savor the here-and-now.

Sometimes the antidote to excessive re-

Acu-points for Reminiscence

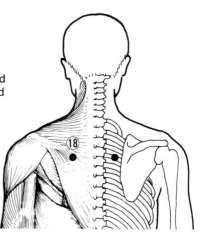

25 : This point was traditionally said to eliminate mental toxicity and "dreams of uncultivated fields."

18 : This point increases self-confidence—i.e., confidence in our present selves and inner Spirits.

Release of all points on the back is also helpful.

miniscence is simply completing the fantasy. Not just reminiscing about the person not married, for instance, up to the point of that decision—and then getting stuck there. Instead, we can complete that fantasy by fantasizing what life with that person might have been like. Not just the "wonderful!" potential, but also all the possible effects upon the evolution and well-being of our body-mind self. Sometimes we then find ourselves remembering our reasons for past choices and actions, rather than just our former dreams.

Reminiscence ceases to control us when we begin to appreciate both the present and the past again. Therefore, as for fear, other antidotes include anything that gets us "out of our heads" and into the here-and-now. If, despite our best efforts, we cannot fully get into the here-and-now, it may be that some aspects of our here-and-now environment need changing.

6. Shock

Shock disturbs the ki and can damage or hurt Shin. Shock, like the other emotions, includes a wide range of experiences of differing intensities. We can be shocked by our income tax bill, or startled when a door bangs shut. We can be even more shocked and traumatized by a threat to our persons or an unpleasant occurrence in the lives of our friends. In extreme conditions, we can literally go into a state of shock—failure in

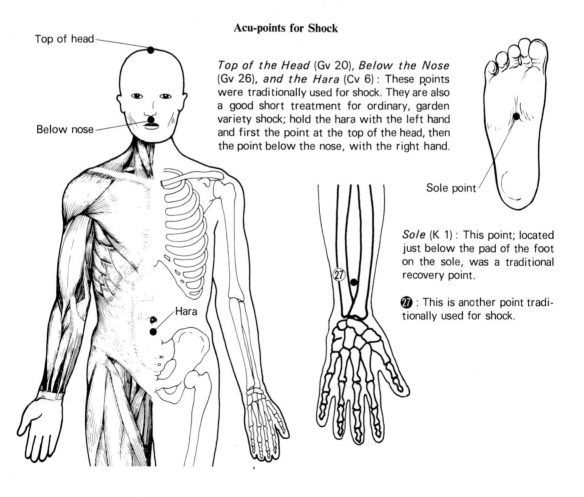

Acu-points for Shock

Top of the Head (Gv 20), *Below the Nose* (Gv 26), *and the Hara* (Cv 6): These points were traditionally used for shock. They are also a good short treatment for ordinary, garden variety shock; hold the hara with the left hand and first the point at the top of the head, then the point below the nose, with the right hand.

Top of head

Below nose

Hara

Sole point

Sole (K 1): This point; located just below the pad of the foot on the sole, was a traditional recovery point.

㉗: This is another point traditionally used for shock.

the circulation of blood.

Some frequency of shocking experiences is almost inherent in modern life. But the frequency seems to be greater if we indulge in too many expectations—projections as to the route that the cycle of change will take, or if we are holding onto a situation, person, or attitude which must be let go of. Therefore, an antidote to run-of-the-mill shock is, again, anything that gets us out of our heads and into the here-and-now present of our entire body-mind selves.

7. Hysteria

Hysteria or over-excitement are states in which Shin is confused and the ki is "suspended at the point of inhalation." We are perpetually "up;" therefore we may crash far down. A general, chronic state of over-excitement may result from "over-pleasure" —a continual search for pleasuse and for the feeling of excitement.

Tuning in to the true desires of the Spirit, listening to our hearts, flowing with the evolutionary cycle of change—these are antidotes to general chronic over-excitement. Just placing the palm over the forehead helps calm the emotional centers. The acu-points given below can be helpful antidotes to a hysterical state of being.

We must not only learn to absorb and circulate ki, but also to tune in to the unity that is our "self" and to find our spiritual center. We must learn to be aware of and release tension almost as soon as it develops, rather than years later. We must experience and appreciate the free flow of ki through our bodies, and therefore also through our "minds"—the emotional, mental, and spiritual aspects of the self. Choosing to allow the vital energy to circulate freely, rather than blocking it up, can be the beginning of learning to really flow with the great river of life— the constant changes that are the very stuff of existence.

Acu-points for Hysteria and Over-excitement

(H 4)
(H 5)
(H 6)
Spirit door
(H 7)

Spirit Door (H 7) : This point helps to balance and calm the heart, residence of Shin, and is helpful for insomnia due to excitement. For hysteria or hysterical reactions, you can simply hold this point and the three points above it (H 6, 5, and 4) with all four fingers, as though you were taking the pulse but on the ulnar side of the hand and with firm pressure.

Base of Skull (Gv 16) *and Center of Sternum* (Cv 17) : These points help to calm the spirit and generally relax the physical and energic condition. You may hold them together, with the right hand on the base of the skull and the left hand on the center of the sternum.

Base of skull

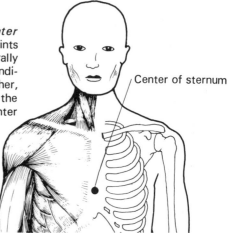
Center of sternum

CONCLUDING THOUGHTS

Giving a Jin Shin Do acupressure treatment is an art. It is an act of creativity proceeding from a feeling of compassion, which unites us with the great cosmic sea of energy. The recipient is, in a sense, an instrument; the energy flows being played and tuned are like the strings of an instrument. But in another sense the recipient is also the creator or artist. For the treater is really just a helper, allowing the recipient to release, balance, and tune himself. Perhaps the main ways in which the treater serves as a helper are through the holding of appropriate acupoints and the channeling of ki; other ways may be through the use of meditation and breathing techniques—as well as through the simple technique of listening.

In all arts, there are these three elements: 1) a vision or feeling which one is expressing or creating; 2) skill in drawing upon the innate potential of the instrument or materials used in that expression; and 3) union with or submersion in the great creative energy. In this union, artist and instrument or materials are partners in the creative act.

The vision of Jin Shin Do is one of body-mind well-being and continual growth. The feeling that Jin Shin Do helps to create is one of freedom, clarity, and flow. The skill is developing the "eye in the fingertips,"—becoming more and more sensitive to the body-mind condition, and becoming freer and more open channels. Union with the universal creative energy is almost synonymous with the art of Jin Shin Do, for it is an inherently meditative technique. This union is strengthened by the processes of hara breathing and channeling.

Art is magic. In Jin Shin Do, the catalyst to the creative act is compassion or love, which is perhaps the highest Magic.

Through Jin Shin Do we can tune into our being in new ways. We can begin to dissolve the body/mind separation in a journey towards the "aware body." We can feel our own specific armored muscular conditions. We can get in touch with our real feelings and dissolve or expel some old emotional states that we have blocked into our physical structures. As the ki begins to flow through the channels and meridians, we can feel this ki flow as a deep state of complete body-mind relaxation. As the regulating channels, or Strange Flows, are unblocked and begin to function freely and harmoniously, we can experience their magical nature—the opening and balancing activities which have given these flows the alternative name "psychic channels." In this process, our physical, emotional, and spiritual natures change, becoming clearer, more centered, and stronger.

Many changes can be felt very quickly. Deep release, balancing, and centering takes time, for it has taken us a long time to develop our body-mind armoring. But even if we could concoct the perfect panacea for immediate, complete, and absolute physical and emotional release and reawakening, it might not even be good for us! Unless awareness develops and deepens, the same problems will return, or be replaced by others. New aspects of the self must be experienced, the boundaries between these aspects must gradually be dissolved, and the unity of our being must be felt. The continual growth of self-awareness is prerequisite for developing or uncovering the freedom, peace, and joy that is our birthright and the potential of our Spirit.

156

Through Jin Shin Do acupressure treatments, through exercise and movement, through diet, and through breathing techniques and meditation, we can become more aware of our body-mind union and of the physical and energic cords uniting us with each other and with the environment.[1] We can reverse the trend of tuning out, begin to erase whatever divisions we have created, and learn to enjoy the whole. We can become more open and free beings, continually growing and unfolding our inner Spirits, and connecting with the Universal Spirit. We do not need to now be or soon become "perfect," but we can be basically happy and free, experiencing the Universal Flow—which is love, which is Magic. This is the Way of Jin Shin Do, the way of the compassionate spirit.

---

[1]Though there is not sufficient space in this volume to go into these aspects of Jin Shin Do, the importance of exercises (both for strengthening and for increasing flexibility) and of a balanced diet cannot be over-estimated.

BIBLIOGRAPHY

In addition to the following books, charts, and reports, a great many verbal sources have been important in the development of Jin Shin Do and of this book. These include teachings and interviews in the areas of: 1) Jin Shin Jitsu and the philosophies of Jiro Murai; 2) acupuncture, including the Chinese, Korean, and Japanese systems; and 3) Taoist yoga techniques and philosophy.

Acupuncture, by Johng Kyo Lee, M.D. and Sang Kook Bae, Kae Chuk Sa Publishing Co., Korea, 1974.

Acupuncture, The Academy Press Co., 57, Wai Ching Street, Kowloon, Hong Kong.

Acupuncture: the Ancient Chinese Art of Healing, by Felix Mann, M.B., Vintage Books, Random House, New York, 1962.

Acupuncture Meridians Chart, by Michimasa Nishizawa, Ichikokan-Ido Laboratory, Japan, 1956.

Acupuncture Vitality, by D. and J. Lawson-Wood, Health Science Press, Rustington, Sussex, England, 1960.

The Art of Glowing Health, by Wen-shan Huang, South Sky Book Co., Hong Kong, 1973.

Atlas Du Meridien Extraordinaire, Japan.

A Barefoot Doctor's Manual, U.S. Department of Health, Education, and Welfare, Public Health Service, National Institute of Health, 1974.

Beyond the Gods—Buddhist & Taoist Mysticism, by John Blofeld, Dutton, N.Y., 1974.

Biorhythm for Health Design, by Kichinosuke Tatai, M.D., M.P.H., Japan Publications, Tokyo and New York, 1977.

Biological Rhythms in Human and Animal Physiology, by Gay Gaerluce, Dover Publications, New York, 1971.

The Book of Macrobiotics: The Universal Way of Health and Happiness, by Michio Kushi, Japan Publications, Tokyo and New York, 1977.

Buddhist Yoga, by Rev. Kanjitsu Iijima, Japan Publications, Tokyo and New York, 1973.

Chinese Acupuncture Medicine, Vol. 2, The Meridian (Pathway) System, by Robert Tsay, M.D. and William W. Shaw, M.D., Association of New Chinese Medicine, Wappinger Falls, N.Y.

The Chinese Art of Healing, by Stephan Palos, Bantam Books, New York, 1971.

Circulus Meridiani Palpabilis et Nomina Punctorum Meridianorum, by Rokurō Fujita, M.D., and Tsutomu Kishi, Kanazawa, Japan.

The Five Elements of Acupuncture and Chinese Massage, by Denis and Joyce Lawson-Wood, Health Science Press, Rustington, Sussex, England, 1965.

Freedom through Cooking, by Iona Teeguarden, Order of the Universe Publications, Boston, 1971.

Journal of the International Congress of Acupuncture and Moxibustion, Japan Acupuncture and Moxibustion Society, Tokyo, 1965.

158

Massage: The Oriental Method, by Katsusuke Serizawa, M.D., Japan Publications, Tokyo and New York, 1972.

The Meridians of Acupuncture, by Felix Mann, M.B., William Heinemann Medical Books Ltd., London, England, 1964.

Meridian Phenomena, by Rokurō Fujita, M.D., Kanazawa, Japan, Ido-no Nippon-sha.

The North American College of Acupuncture textbook, by Kok Leung, Portland, Oregon.

An Outline of Chinese Acupuncture, by the Academy of Traditional Chinese Medicine, Foreign Languages Press, Peking, 1975.

Principles of Chinese Acupuncture Medicine, by David C. Chu, DCM and PhD, and Dorothy W. Chu, AB and MT, Rainbow Printing Ltd., Hong Kong.

Psychic Discoveries Behind the Iron Curtain, by Sheila Ostrander and Lynn Schroeder, Bantam Books, New York, 1970.

Psychoenergetic Systems, An International Journal, edited by Stanley Krippner, Gordon and Breach Science Publishers Ltd., Great Britain, 1976.

The Secret and the Sublime: Taoist Mysteries and Magic, by John Blofeld, Dutton, New York, 1973.

The Secret of the Golden Flower, by Richard Wilhelm, translator, Harcourt, Brace, and World, Inc., New York, 1962.

Shiatsu: Japanese Finger-pressure Therapy, by Tokujiro Namikoshi, Japan Publications, Tokyo and New York, 1972.

Shiatsu Therapy: Theory and Practice, by Toru Namikoshi, Japan Publications, Tokyo and New York, 1974.

The Taoist Art of Radiant Health, manuscript by Sung Jin Park.

Taoist Health Exercise Book, by Da Liu, Links Books, New York, 1974.

Tao Te Ching, a New Translation by Ch'u Ta-Kao, George Allen and Unwin Ltd., London, England, 1937.

Tao: the Watercourse Way, by Alan Watts with Al Chung-liang Huang, Pantheon Books, Random House, New York, 1975.

The Theoretical Foundations of Chinese Medicine, by Manfred Porkett, M.I.T. Press, Cambridge, Massachusetts, 1974.

Treatment of Acupuncture, by So Tin Yau, Kowloon, Hong Kong.

The Treatment of Disease by Acupuncture, by Felix Mann, William Heinemann Medical Books Ltd., London, England, 1963.

Tsubo: Vital Points for Oriental Therapy, by Katsusuke Serizawa, M.D., Japan Publications, Tokyo and New York, 1976.

The Yellow Emperor's Classic of Internal Medicine (Huang Ti Nei Ching Su Wen), translated by Ilza Veith, University of California Press, Berkeley 1970.

Zen Shiatsu: How to Harmonize Yin and Yang for Better Health, by Shizuto Masunaga with Wataru Ohashi and the Shiatsu Education Center of America, Japan Publications, Tokyo and New York, 1977.